OMEGA 3 CUISINE

recipes for
health and pleasure

by

Alan Roettinger
with Udo Erasmus

books
Alive

Summertown,
Tennessee

Pictured on the cover:
Vegetable Lasagne, page 166

Cover design: Paul Gregory Newman
Front cover and interior photos: Warren Jefferson
Interior design: Gwynelle Dismukes
Food styling: Alan Roettinger

Published by Books Alive
P.O. Box 99
Summertown, TN 38483
1-888-260-8458
www.bookpubco.com

Printed in Canada

ISBN 978-0-920470-81-7

16   15   14   13   12   11   10   09   08   10 9 8 7 6 5 4 3 2

Library of Congress Cataloging-in-Publication Data

Roettinger, Alan, 1952-
  Omega-3 cuisine : recipes for health and pleasure / by Alan Roettinger ; with Udo Erasmus.
      p. cm.
  Includes index.
   ISBN 978-0-920470-81-7
  1. High-omega-3 fatty acid diet--Recipes. I. Erasmus, Udo. II. Title.
  RM237.62.R64 2008
  641.5'6384--dc22
                                     2008001436

Books Alive is a member of Green Press Initiative. We chose to print this title on paper with postconsumer recycled content, processed without chlorine, which saved the following natural resources:

15 tons of wood
4,776 lbs of solid waste
37,188 gallons of water
8,959 lbs of greenhouse gases
71 million BTU

For more information, visit <www.greenpressinitiative.org>. Savings calculations thanks to the Environmental Defense Paper Calculator, <www.papercalculator.org>.

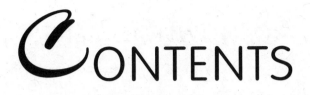

CONTENTS

Acknowledgments

I'm a thief. Every chef is. All of us begin with elements and ideas we pick up from other chefs. That's one reason so many chefs are insecure and jealously guard their recipes. My feeling has always been, go ahead—take my recipe and do your best with it. Why? Because I know that every cook brings something unique to the dish, something that's not in the recipe, whether it's an ingredient added, a shortcut taken, a personal technique used, or just an attitude, a feeling. That makes my food securely matchless, regardless of what I've stolen from other chefs or what other chefs steal from me. Inevitably, I will monkey with what I use as a starting point, bending, stretching, altering, adding, and taking away, until the dish is mine. This will be true for you too, believe me, even if you set out to duplicate exactly what I've done. This is a good thing.

I never trained formally under anyone. However, as a self-taught chef I have to acknowledge all the great men and women from whom I not only stole many ideas and foundational recipes, but derived tremendous inspiration. Although I've only met and cooked with a very few of them, their influence in my cooking is undeniable, and I owe my success to their generosity in sharing their techniques, opinions, dedication to excellence, and, yes, their recipes. Most inspiring to me are Jacques Pépin, Bobby Hendry, Titi Benoffi, Jeremiah Tower, Fredy Girardet, Charlie Trotter, Joachim Splichal, Georges Blanc, Alice Medrich, Emily Luchetti, and collectively, too numerous to name, the hundreds whose food I have enjoyed, knowing full well the hard work that went into every single detail. Hats off to all of them.

Preface

Health is a state of being—our natural state of being. It is the direct, unencumbered relationship between life and the body. Health comes from life. Life, the energy that keeps us alive—and that separates from the body at the time of death—is health. It cannot get sick, cannot deteriorate, and cannot die. Life created the genetic program—our DNA—that serves as the blueprint for body construction, maintenance, and repair. Our genetic program was made by life within nature, and was made for life in nature.

Life determines which molecules are the essential building blocks of the body: minerals, vitamins, essential amino acids from proteins, and essential fatty acids (EFAs) from the right kinds of fats. If we want optimum health, we need optimum intake of these essential building blocks in an undamaged form. Life didn't supply us with a blueprint for making these essential nutrients. They must therefore be supplied from outside the body, through foods or supplements.

Life also determines which molecules are poisons to the body. Foremost among these are man-made synthetic molecules, which have never been present in nature. Life has not yet developed effective ways of counteracting, neutralizing, or getting rid of them. By changing the way our genes perform, many different kinds of synthetic molecules can turn our genetic program for health into a program for disease. Among the synthetic molecules that can have negative effects on health are pesticides, plastics, industrial chemicals, pharmaceutical drugs, and food molecules damaged by industry through processing. Also, we may damage food molecules unknowingly through our own food preparation and storage methods.

Healthcare involves protecting and nourishing our natural state of being through proper nutrition, exercise, relationships, and inspiration. Practicing good healthcare enables us to enjoy long, active, pain-free lives. When we ignore any component of healthcare, especially for extended periods, our health is compromised, resulting in disease, pain, and a shortened life span.

Life itself is health, complete and inviolable. The body, on the other hand, is always under construction. And a major construction site it is, even when it is not diseased. About 98 percent of the molecules in the body are removed and replaced every year. That's why we must eat, drink, breathe, sleep, and clean the body on a regular basis, all of which take continuous attention and effort.

The upside of the fact that the body is always under major construction, renovation, and repair is that healing is possible. By making the appropriate changes in the kinds of foods we eat, how we prepare them, how we eat them, and how we fashion our lifestyle, we can rebuild 98 percent of a diseased body into a healthy body. That is very good news.

Healing, then, depends in large part on changes we make in the way we eat, which in turn, depend on the way we think and feel. Healing also depends on the environment we choose to live in and the influences we allow ourselves to be exposed to. It's easy to see how living in a polluted environment may negatively affect our health, but we may overlook the stress factors introduced by overexposure to depressing news, for example, or to violent images in films. Unsatisfactory or abusive relationships can also impede the healing process.

Most importantly, healing depends on how close we are to life itself. Life is not only the source of physical health; it is also the source of mental and emotional health. Life, the power behind our breath, is the source of joy. Staying close to that power in our awareness is the surest way to enjoy our life and ensure that the engine of healing runs smoothly. Feelings of love, gratitude, and contentment abound when we are in touch with life. Although there are myriad factors that affect and influence physical health, no one has ever had a heart attack or been stricken with cancer from feeling too much gratitude, joy, or peace.

In order to set the stage for physical healing to occur, it is crucial that we understand one thing: we must make changes in the way we eat. Not only must we do this for healing, we must do it for ongoing health. Clearly, we must not revert to our former ways of eating once the symptoms of disease diminish or disappear, unless we wish for them to recur.

Except for humans and the animals that depend on humans for food, every creature that has ever lived has eaten all its food fresh, whole, raw, and organic. That is nature's food standard. When we cook food, we depart from nature's food standard. The harsher the cooking method, the further we depart from nature's standard. Cooking over steam is better than cooking in water, which is much better than sautéing in oil, which in turn is vastly better than deep-frying. If food is free of bacterial or other toxic microorganisms, raw food is better than food that has been cooked.

Because cooked food has become a standard of virtually every modern cuisine, most people have become accustomed to eating their food prepared this way. Unfortunately, our physiology has not adapted to the loss of essential nutrients and other components of health that are present only in raw foods. Therefore, I am a strong proponent of using digestive enzymes with meals to replace the enzymes in food that are destroyed by cooking.

I also recommend brushing teeth with probiotics at the end of a meal to replace the beneficial bacteria that were killed when the food was cooked. I advocate using supplements to replace minerals that are leached out of food and vitamins that are destroyed during cooking. I have found them to be very helpful. When I follow these practices, I experience less pain, have more energy, and feel better all around.

Finally, I advise against using oils for cooking. Oils contain the most sensitive of the essential nutrients that life requires us to eat. They are easily destroyed and can easily be made toxic by exposure to light, air, and heat. In the frying pan, oils are made toxic by the simultaneous effects of all three of these destructive influences. The recipes in this book are designed to avoid overheating oils. They are beneficial for our health because they follow the standards of good physical health set by life.

Just as good nutrition and health are related, poor nutrition and disease are related. By eating foods that promote the body's functions and build healthy tissue—prepared in ways that protect the food's nutrients—we may enjoy optimum physical health. If we eat foods that interfere with the body's functions or damage its tissues, disease is sure to follow. It's important to also note that even good food can be rendered harmful when prepared in ways that alter its natural state; the more radically food is altered (as with burning), the greater the harm. This cannot be overstated!

Once our health has been compromised, whether by a lapse of healthcare or by external influences, such as viruses or injuries, we may require medical intervention. Not to be confused with healthcare, the practice of medicine is the treatment of disease and, in some cases, the application of preventive measures.

Unfortunately, the instruction doctors receive in medical school relates primarily to disease, with an emphasis on treatment; they only get a cursory peek at the subject of nutrition. Consequently, doctors' understanding of health revolves around the many things that can go wrong and the strategies to contain, reverse, or repair health problems. Fortunately, more doctors today are taking it upon themselves to continue their education in nutrition; some even investigate the effectiveness of alternative therapies, such as acupuncture. However, no doctor and no treatment can take the place of our own commitment to be responsible for maintaining our health.

Contrary to popular misconception, drugs have nothing to do with the natural state called health. There are a number of lifesaving substances, such as insulin and bioidentical thyroid hormone, that allow people with certain conditions to live normal lives they otherwise would not, but these are the exception, not the rule. Nutrients are the building blocks of a healthy body. Drugs are not. Drugs provide disease management, symptom suppression, crisis intervention, and life-support systems. Although many drugs are either derivatives or synthetic forms of compounds from plants found in nature, they contain unnatural molecules. Their side effects confirm that they do not belong in a healthy human body. They are tools for crisis management only and should be considered a measure of last resort.

It is important to make the distinction between healthcare, which is the individual's responsibility, and medicine, for which one is dependent upon physicians. If we take care of our health, the need for medical intervention will not come up often; if we ignore or abuse our health, medical intervention may become a constant need—and an expensive one. It's a good idea to have regular physical exams in order to make sure your body is working properly and no problems are developing. But it is equally important to take charge of your own health and observe healthy habits to maintain it.

Inspired people who love life apply nutrition and lifestyle as the interventions of choice. Inspiration is also a key factor in health. When we are inspired, we feel energetic. When we feel energetic, we can easily do the necessary work to maintain our health. Then our bodies function at their highest possible level. Our posture is better, we have even more energy, and our choices of food, recreation, relationships, and work are more likely to benefit our health and our life.

The immune system is enhanced when we are inspired, just as it is weakened if we become depressed. The best option for people who want to enjoy their life to the fullest is to be inspired so that they have the energy to take responsibility for the care of their health.

Inspired people quite naturally feel empowered to take on the challenge and responsibility of maintaining their health. They're able to live in line with nature because they have a choice. This is a major difference between diseased and healthy people. I highly recommend that you look within and become inspired by the wonder of life, by the miracle of breath and the feeling of contentment at the core of your being. Be thrilled by the unimaginable genius that transformed a handful of dust and three buckets of water into the beautiful body you inhabit—the amazing, automatic way in which lettuce is turned into toenails, potatoes into eyeballs, and everything you eat into what is your body, from your toenails to your eyeballs.

Life, using a genetic program it created, transforms the creatures of nature that you eat into your profoundly astonishing body with all of its cells (60 trillion of them!), tissues (256 at last count), glands, and organs, making it possible for dust and water to have the human experience. To live, breathe, laugh, cry, sing, see, hear, feel, dance, think, talk, grow, heal, love, perform, master, and as if that's not marvelous enough, even reproduce, has got to be the greatest miracle in the world.

Looking for a miracle? Go check yourself out in a mirror. You're it! There is no greater miracle than you, alive and kickin'. How inspiring is that?

Udo Erasmus, PhD

INTRODUCTION

We eat for many reasons. Obviously, we need to eat for survival, but there is much more to it than that. We also eat for comfort, pleasure, and entertainment. We eat to celebrate and socialize, to impress, and to network with business associates. Some of us eat to try to compensate for a sense of lack or in response to unresolved emotional problems.

We hunger on many levels, and we eat as part of an ongoing attempt to fulfill ourselves. Some of our eating is helpful to our quest for fulfillment, and some of our eating is detrimental to it. Herein lies a puzzle that anyone who wishes to enjoy a healthy, fulfilling life must unravel and individually resolve.

Chefs in this day and age often find themselves struggling with the mixed challenge of offering their clientele interesting fare, packed with flavor, and at least some pretense of its being healthful. Catch phrases like "low fat," "all natural," "low carb," and "high fiber" are thrown around liberally in the hope that customers will feel good about what they are eating.

The food industry's attempt is to create an appearance of something wholesome, while serving up a product that thrills the palate, surprises the imagination, gratifies the stomach, and still generates a decent profit. That's a tall order, so it should come as no surprise that somewhere along the line compromises are inevitably made. Given the burden of attracting business, garnering fame, and making money, guess where the corners will be cut. That's right—your health. It's not that anyone sets out to harm the client—that would be self-defeating—but restaurants and food manufacturers are in it to make money. Whether or not what they offer is actually all that good for you is largely irrelevant.

Part of the problem is that many chefs, if not most, have poor eating habits themselves, stemming from a lack of basic nutritional information along with inescapably ingrained attitudes handed down by generations of great cooks who have always favored flavor and pleasure over health and longevity. The purpose of this book is to bring flavor and health together so that there need be no trade-off on either end.

In order for food to be truly health promoting it must appeal to the senses. It's a well-established fact that digestion begins with an appetizing thought, sight, aroma, or taste. If what you contemplate eating is appealing to your senses, your digestive juices will begin flowing even before the first bite is taken.

Unfortunately, there is often a considerable rift between what we perceive as good food and what our body can successfully process to our ultimate benefit. The result is that although we may like the thought, sight, smell, and taste of something, consuming it could bring us undesirable consequences, such as indigestion, acid reflux, obesity, chronic fatigue, diabetes, cardiovascular disease, or cancer.

Think about how it happens. First you feel a little hungry. At this point, you just want to eat something. If nothing is presented to you right then, your mind will begin to generate ideas about what to eat. If you are in the habit of making poor food choices, such as highly refined carbohydrates and fried food, your mind will likely conjure up images of these foods in response to your hunger. If someone were to suggest a more wholesome alternative (like a salad instead of doughnuts or french fries), there is a good chance you would not be swayed by it. Your mind is hooked on something it recalls as satisfying, and only that sort of something will do.

Note that it's never the mind that's hungry; it's the body. Quite unfairly, the mind gets to decide what will be eaten, while the onerous task of digesting it will be relegated entirely to the body. In the aftermath of every dietary indiscretion, the mind flits merrily off to its next virtual adventure—which may even include tormenting you for making poor choices. Meanwhile, the body is left with all the work.

How to reverse this phenomenon? Begin by paying attention to the way you feel. Don't worry about what you're eating just yet—simply observe what happens after you eat. Is your body happy with what just came down, or is it already plotting revenge? Do you feel light and full of energy or heavy and sluggish? Are your eyes clear or red and slightly glazed? Are your sinuses open or clogged? Are you burping up the flavors of something you ate two meals ago? These signs and symptoms are the lexicon of the body—the only means it has to communicate with you. Pay close attention.

Once you've begun to recognize the messages your body is sending you, and you are able to match them up with the action that prompted them, you're ready to begin retraining your desires. This is going to take a little time, so don't be too concerned about your progress. Just start eating according to Udo's recommendations and see how you feel. Be especially attentive when you deviate or revert to your "normal" way of eating.

One word of caution: When you first begin eating a lot of salad and raw foods, you may experience some gas. Believe it or not, this is normal. Raw foods are high in natural fiber, which acts like a broom—in effect, scrubbing out the digestive tract. Most people who have been subsisting on highly processed foods will experience a period of cleansing when they switch to a diet of raw food and complex carbohydrates. Give it a week or two before you take the presence of gas as a negative sign. Don't worry, it'll pass. (Sorry—I couldn't resist.)

The recipes in this book will be a valuable resource in your effort to change your eating habits. They have all been created with the senses in mind, meaning that enjoyment is a key factor. Reading them should spark images of interesting, appetizing dishes. I'm not out to convince anyone to eat unappealing "health food." Whereas Udo's area of expertise is health and well-being, mine is flavor and the pleasure of eating. I could never "eat healthy" if it meant I had to hold my nose and suffer through some awful-tasting, weird-textured, hippie fodder. To me, if it doesn't taste good, it isn't food. The Creator wisely put taste buds and olfactory receptors at the entrance to our digestive tract so we could enjoy what we eat; the exit was very kindly placed behind us, out of sight, sans taste buds, at a relatively safe distance from the nose. If it were the other way around, we probably would starve to death.

I set about learning Udo's Right Fat Diet precepts and devised recipes that adhere to them. So all you have to do is choose whichever dishes appeal to you and start cooking. As you'll notice, nothing in this book is cooked in a manner that will result in caramelization or browning. Udo refers to this as "burned food," which is to say that it is chemically altered to the point that it has ceased to be something your body can assimilate properly and, if eaten, will be injurious to your health. In these recipes, when ingredients are heated in a small amount of oil, some water or wine is often added to prevent this from happening. In some cases, a recipe will instruct you to "sweat" the vegetables, which is done over very low heat, with a lid in place to keep the moisture contained. This process is similar to sautéing but does not color the vegetables. It's important to check on the food from time to time so you get the desirable flavor enrichment without "burning" it.

In every recipe where heating occurs, Udo's Oil is added *after* the procedure is completed and the food has been removed from the heat source. Even though the oil will be warmed by the food, it will not be overheated. This way, the molecular integrity of the oil will not be damaged and the beneficial properties will remain intact.

I know the points I've raised represent a hard-line philosophy regarding diet and cooking that may seem rather extreme. Maybe you're thinking that becoming more conscious of what you eat will make dining out less exciting. But if you knew what I know about what goes on behind the kitchen door in restaurants, then what I've laid out would be the least of your concerns.

Now, I'm not advocating a paranoid, isolationist, Howard Hughes–type worldview. I travel, and I enjoy eating out on occasion. I'm merely suggesting that you minimize your exposure to food of questionable origin that is prepared with profit, not your health, in mind. Regardless of your level of culinary expertise, once you understand what's good for you, the best food you'll ever get will be on your plate when you cook and eat at home.

Alan Roettinger

THE RIGHT FAT DIET

In his book entitled Fats That Heal, Fats That Kill Udo Erasmus points out in great detail that there are good fats, which we must have for optimum health, and there are bad fats, which we need to avoid if we wish to prevent degenerative diseases and premature death. His book is the definitive volume on fats and their relationship to health, offering a wealth of information—both in molecular terms, which is of interest to the scientifically minded, and in accessible layman's terms. Reading this book is highly recommended for anyone with a keen interest in health. The intention behind this chapter is to offer you just a few salient points, which may serve as an introduction to the fats recommended in this cookbook and why they are of particular importance.

For many years, fat has unfairly suffered a bad reputation. People interested in enjoying good health, keeping a slim figure, and avoiding heart problems have been told again and again to drastically reduce their intake of fat. To many, this might seem like common sense—if you don't want to *be* fat, don't *eat* fat. But there is a lot more to the relationship between fats and health than that.

There are two separate issues to consider: looks and health. Although these often go hand in hand, they just as often do not. For many people, the outward appearance of health—a slim, attractive body—is central to their sense of well-being. While understandable, this view is rather limited, and in terms of one's health, somewhat misguided. Naturally, we all want to look good. However, there are many conditions of poor health that may not manifest in our appearance until they have reached very advanced, even life-threatening stages.

The Right Fat Diet, while helpful in maintaining one's optimum weight, is not merely about appearances; it's about what's going on inside, and providing the body with the best building blocks to keep it all in good working order. Good fats are central to this diet, because although they are essential to our health and well-being, incredibly, most of us don't get enough of them.

Since looks remain a primary concern for people, let's get that out of the way first. The common assumption that being overweight is the result of eating too much fat is erroneous. Eating excessive fat, especially saturated fat, or literally any refined, overheated, or hydrogenated fat, is harmful to health in a number of ways, which we'll come to next. But obesity itself is the result of eating an excess of carbohydrates, especially highly refined "white food," such as white sugar, white flour, and white rice.

What constitutes "excessive" in terms of carbohydrates? Simple: it's any amount we ingest but do not immediately use for fuel. The more refined the carbohydrate, the faster we need to begin the process of burning it (as with strenuous exercise) in order to prevent the body from storing it as fat. Brown rice (a complex carbohydrate), for example, takes longer to break down than pasta made from refined durum wheat. Whereas pasta is ready-to-burn starch, brown rice contains a considerable amount of fiber, protein, fat, and minerals. If we don't want that spaghetti to become part of our waistline, we'll need to get up from the table right away and do some serious working out. Complex carbohydrates—whole grains, beans, and starchy vegetables—take longer for the body to sort out, buying us some time before the starches (sugars) are ready to be either burned for energy or converted to fat. Fruits, though high in sugar, are generally problematic only when consumed in large quantities and in a high ratio to the other foods we eat. The bottom line: any carbohydrates we eat but don't use by the time our body has them processed and available for fuel will become that dreaded, unattractive flab.

Sadly, once the sugars in our food have been converted to fat for later use as fuel, they cannot be converted back to sugars (such as glucose, a principal fuel used by the brain). That fat is only good for grunt work, and only after we have used up new fuel (from the food we just ate) will the stored fat begin to burn. Anyone who has tried to lose weight by exercise alone knows how hard it is to reach that fat-burning threshold.

So, if you're trying to lose weight, you have to eliminate simple sugars and refined carbohydrates from your diet, eat protein, essential fats, and leafy vegetables, and get a lot of strenuous exercise. The good news is, by following this regimen you'll also be headed for better overall health.

The most important thing to avoid is refined food, because not only is it rapidly digested (and turned into fat), it also has been stripped of essential nutrients and fiber, so it is nutritionally worthless. Refined food is a modern invention, known originally only to the affluent classes, who could afford the labor-intensive processing involved in turning whole grains into white flour and sugarcane into white sugar. It wasn't until the industrial revolution that refining procedures became economical for mass production. Commercial products that deliver these refined foods to the masses are an even more recent development.

The emergence of degenerative disease as a major scourge can be directly traced to the proliferation of refined food products, especially refined oils. Where once obesity, cardiovascular disease, and cancer affected primarily the aristocracy, today anyone can afford to eat refined food, live a sedentary lifestyle, and be similarly afflicted. This is the butt end of what we loosely refer to as "progress."

The understanding that refined carbohydrates are the cause of obesity (and not fats per se) has only lately begun to take root. We now know that Dr. Atkins (may his portly self rest in peace) was right about one thing: carbohydrates make you fat, not fats. The problem with his diet system was that he didn't differentiate between good fats and bad fats. A slim, attractive person can be just as unhealthy as a fat, unattractive person. Girth is only one factor among many that can affect your health, and only one of the more obvious indicators. A svelte figure may improve your self-esteem (and possibly your social acceptance), but unless you've accomplished this by eating nutritious food and exercising regularly, it will eventually come back to bite that bony little sit-upon you've worked so hard to cultivate.

The heart of the Right Fat Diet is optimizing our intake of good fats while eliminating bad fats, which is based on an understanding of the effect that both of these fats have on our health. Of all the fats we eat, only certain omega-3 and omega-6 fats are essential nutrients; this means that our body is not able to make them from other nutrients we consume and must obtain them from our diet directly. Every single cell in the human body needs and uses these fats. They are absolutely necessary in order for the body to function properly, prevent degenerative diseases, and avoid premature death. Most people get enough omega-6 fats in their diet—although for the most part, not from good sources—but an estimated 99 percent of the population gets insufficient omega-3s.

> A single tablespoon of oil that is 1 percent process–damaged may contain as many as 60,000,000,000,000,000,000,000 damaged molecules. Think about it . . . That's over a million unnatural *(and toxic)* molecules for each one of your body's 60 trillion cells!

Research shows that four of the major degenerative conditions of our time—cancer, cardiovascular disease, diabetes, and arthritis—improve when our intake of omega-3 fats increases, which is a clear indication that these conditions are caused at least in part by omega-3 deficiency.

Obtaining essential fats from our diet is important enough, but it's not the whole story. If our body is to absorb and put these fats to good use for optimum health, they must come to us free of pesticides, synthetic chemicals, and damaged molecules. The first two pollutants (pesticides and synthetic chemicals) are easy to avoid simply by obtaining our healthful fats from organically grown nuts and seeds. Avoiding damaged molecules is somewhat more problematic because fats, especially omega-3s, are sensitive to injury by heat, light, and oxygen, which are unavoidable in the standard commercial methods of extracting, refining, bleaching, and deodorizing oils. With the exception of extra-virgin olive oil, virtually all of the bottles of oil on supermarket shelves contain process-damaged molecules.

Producing healthful fats for consumption is no small feat. First, the extraction method must not expose the fats to high heat, light, or oxygen. Second, the oils obtained must not be "refined"—a destructive process involving harsh chemicals (caustic soda, phosphoric acid, and bleaching clays) and further heating (literally to frying temperatures)—which is done to give oils a longer shelf life, but it also effectively removes much of their nutritional value and damages some of their molecules. These altered molecules have never existed in nature, so our body is not prepared to deal with them, let alone utilize them as nutrients. Oils produced this way are worse than merely useless, however; they are in fact toxic to our system, causing inflammation, cardiovascular disease, and cancer.

Dark Glass vs. Dark Plastic

Synthetic chemicals will leach into any liquid stored in plastic, which accounts for the odd taste we may detect when drinking water from a plastic bottle. Oils swell plastic, enhancing this leaching action. That's in clear plastic, which is bad enough, but in order to protect so-called "cold-pressed" oil from light, some producers store it in dark plastic bottles. The pigment used to darken the plastic, called furnace black, is known to contain carcinogenic molecules. In my opinion, these plastic containers in particular should really come with a skull and crossbones warning on them! The way to avoid contamination by toxic chemicals is to store all liquids, especially oils, in glass containers.

It's not enough to avoid overheating the fats; the extraction method must also protect fats from light and oxygen. Provided this method is in place, and provided the oil is not refined, three steps remain to ensure that fats will reach the consumer in a healthful condition. First, the container must provide protection from light, oxygen, and contamination. Second, the container itself must not introduce contaminants (such as synthetic chemicals, which are present in plastic). Third, it must be stored refrigerated to protect the oil from heat and keep it from deteriorating, since no refining steps have been taken to extend its shelf life. This is a very tall order, so manufacturers of commercial oils have their work cut out for them if they are going to meet the challenge of producing and marketing healthful fats.

In 1983, after extensive study, Udo began pioneering a new technology for extracting oils from seeds with nutrition and health in mind rather than shelf life and profit. The system he developed includes low-heat pressing and also provides protection of the oils from light and oxygen. Because he had entered the field with an interest in healing and health, all of the results he sought were centered on what works, not on what sells. Since that time, Udo has consistently worked to set the highest possible standard for health and nutrition in general, and for fats in particular.

Udo's Oil 3•6•9 Blend offers a truly healthful source of undamaged essential fats in the right proportion of omega-3 to omega-6 for maximum health benefits. It comes to market in a dark glass bottle, flushed with nitrogen to exclude oxygen, packaged in a cardboard box for further protection from light, and refrigerated.

In recent years, a lot of media attention has been given to the benefits of fish oil, a rich source of the omega-3 derivative DHA. Because DHA is necessary for the development and function of nerve cells in the brain and eyes, and because omega-3 fatty acids in general are lacking in the diet of most people, many doctors recommend fish oil supplements highly. Unfortunately for vegetarians and vegans, fish oil is not an option as a DHA supplement.

The good news is that Udo's Oil now offers a vegan source of DHA derived from microalgae (the same place the fish get it) grown in contaminant-free tanks. Labeled Udo's Oil DHA Blend, this DHA oil is combined with the same essential fats as the 3•6•9 blend, produced with the same standards of health and quality. Whenever Udo's Oil is called for in a recipe in this book, use either Udo's Oil 3•6•9 Blend or Udo's Oil DHA 3•6•9 Blend, whichever you prefer.

It's a well-known fact that fats enhance food flavors, which is why we enjoy eating fatty food. Here are some other facts that may not be as well-known:

☞ *Good* fats actually help burn body fat!

☞ *Good* fats improve digestion and reduce cravings for sugar and other carbohydrates.

☞ *Good* fats improve the absorption of oil-soluble nutrients into the body.

☞ *Good* fats increase energy level and lift mood.

☞ *Good* fats speed healing, increase stamina, and improve focus and performance.

How's *that* for good news!

Infused Oils

Our main objective in this cookbook is to incorporate Udo's Oil into a wide range of dishes in ways that enrich your enjoyment of food while delivering the desired healthful qualities of much-needed essential fatty acids (EFAs). An ideal starting point for this is infusion. The recipes in this chapter involve a simple process by which oil is imbued with flavor, aroma, and color. Once infused, the oil can then enhance other recipes by contributing to the taste, smell, and eye appeal of the finished dish.

Several companies now produce oils infused with various flavors, such as basil or garlic. Commercially, where the health benefits are not considered paramount (if at all), infusion is accomplished by heating the oil with various aromatics. In order to protect the fragile qualities of Udo's Oil, the same results will be obtained without heating, in some cases by increasing the quantity of the flavoring agents. The procedure is quite simple, as you will see. Oil has a marvelous propensity for absorbing flavor from ingredients that are placed in it, especially ingredients that are naturally high in oil, like hot chiles. No doubt you'll find dozens of applications once you get accustomed to preparing and using infused oils.

Bear in mind that most of the aromatics that will be released into the oil are very fragile, especially those derived from fresh herbs. Once infused, the oil should be used as soon as possible. If you want a good variety of flavors but can't use the oils up quickly, it's best to store them in the freezer, where they will keep for up to one month. Use dark glass bottles to protect the fragile essential fats from light. Remember that in order to prevent the leaching of nasty chemicals into the oils, they should never be stored in plastic!

Simple Garlic Oil

Makes about 1 cup

4 to 7 cloves garlic (see note)
1 cup Udo's Oil

Pass the garlic cloves through a garlic press into a small jar. Add the oil and stir. Pour into a clean glass jar or bottle. Simple Garlic Oil will keep for about 1 week in the refrigerator or 1 month in the freezer.

> Adjust the number of garlic cloves to fewer than 4 or more than 7, according to your taste.

Basil Oil

Makes about 1 cup

2½ cups fresh basil leaves, packed
1 cup Udo's Oil

Blanch the basil in boiling water for 15 seconds, drain, and immediately plunge into ice water to stop the cooking completely. Chop coarsely and squeeze out the excess water. Combine the basil in a blender with the oil and process for 2 to 3 minutes, until the mixture turns bright green. Refrigerate for 8 to 12 hours. Strain through several layers of cheesecloth and return to the refrigerator.

Use the oil as is, or allow it to settle for a few hours and then decant to a clean bottle, discarding any residue that has gathered at the bottom of the container. Basil Oil will keep for about 1 week in the refrigerator or 1 month in the freezer.

What could be easier? If you like garlic, this will immediately become a staple in your kitchen. It's the quickest and easiest oil infusion, requiring no straining, decanting, or any other monkeying around. Properly steamed vegetables really need nothing else. Merely drizzle some of this oil on them and you will have a dish that anyone will eat with pleasure. It'll turn pedestrian mashed potatoes into something truly special. Keep some of this on hand in your refrigerator and you'll discover countless uses for it. It's a standard ingredient in many of the recipes in this book.

This is a deliciously fragrant oil, which you can use to impart a vibrant dash of flavor and color as a finishing touch to any number of dishes. It adds depth and complexity to salad dressings and combines particularly well with fresh tomatoes.

Chili Oil

Makes about 1 cup

12 dried red chiles, stems removed
1 cup Udo's Oil

*P*lace the chiles in a small bowl and cover with boiling water. Let sit for about 15 minutes, until the chiles are softened. Drain and pat dry with paper towels. Combine the chiles in a blender with the oil and process for 2 to 3 minutes, until thoroughly blended.

Refrigerate for 8 to 12 hours. Strain through several layers of cheesecloth and return to the refrigerator. After 24 hours, decant to a clean bottle, discarding any residue that has gathered at the bottom of the container.

If you like spicy food keep a small bottle of this in your refrigerator and you will always have a vibrant additive for any dish that needs a love bite. If you're not yet enamored with the fragrant sting of hot chiles, try adding more, not less. Eventually your body will send a signal to your brain requesting an opiate to dull the burn. The body will release endorphins, slowly flooding your system with a pleasant euphoria. Eventually, the flavor, the burn, and a floating bliss will meld together deliciously. Once you reach that endorphin plateau, you'll be a lifelong convert!

This infusion is fairly stable. Stored in the refrigerator, Chili Oil will keep until the expiration date of the Udo's Oil. If you want a spicier oil, add more chiles. If you want a redder color but not much more heat, break open the additional chiles first and remove the seeds.

Curry Oil

Makes about 1 cup

¼ cup almond oil (see note)

1 teaspoon whole cumin seeds

1 teaspoon whole coriander seeds

1 stick cinnamon

2 bay leaves

2 dried red chiles (optional)

2 shallots, finely chopped

2 tablespoons peeled and chopped fresh ginger

1 tablespoon chopped garlic

3 tablespoons curry powder

1 teaspoon sea salt

1 cup Udo's Oil

*P*lace the almond oil in a small saucepan. Add the cumin and coriander seeds, cinnamon stick, bay leaves, and optional chiles, and place over very low heat to warm the oil and release the aromatics of the spices. Add the shallots, ginger, and garlic and stir for 2 minutes longer. Add the curry powder and salt and stir until all the ingredients are thoroughly saturated with the oil. Do not overheat or allow any of the ingredients to brown! Remove from the heat and let the mixture cool completely.

Stir in the Udo's Oil, combining it well. Pour into a glass container and refrigerate for 8 to 12 hours. Strain through several layers of cheesecloth and decant to a clean bottle. Curry Oil will keep for about 1 week in the refrigerator or 1 month in the freezer.

Curry is probably an entirely British creation, invented to enable the uninitiated to imitate the vastly varied cuisine of India. Fortunately, Indian food is so majestic that somehow the power of the original cuisine manages to shine through even this crude effrontery. Curry powder, while falling pathetically short of true Indian flavor, allows even the least experienced cook to add a unique and complex taste to virtually any dish, rendering it, shall we say, *reminiscent* of Indian food. Go for it—it's one of the most useful oils in this section.

Almond oil offers the most neutral taste of all the unrefined oils. It is used in mayonnaise and similar recipes where the taste of Udo's Oil alone would overpower the other flavors. In Ayurvedic medicine, almond oil is considered beneficial to the brain and nervous system. It is also an anti-inflammatory and helpful to the immune system. I use Flora brand almond oil, which is produced by the same exacting standards as Udo's Oil. Look for it in the refrigerated section of natural food stores.

Herb Oil

Makes about 1 cup

    1 cup watercress
    ½ cup snipped chives
    ½ cup fresh parsley
    ¼ cup fresh tarragon
    1 cup Udo's Oil

*B*lanch the herbs in boiling water for 15 seconds, drain, and immediately plunge into ice water to stop the cooking completely. Chop coarsely and squeeze out the excess water. Combine the herbs in a blender with the oil and process for about 2 minutes, until bright green. Refrigerate for 8 to 12 hours. Strain through several layers of cheesecloth and return to the refrigerator.

Use the oil as is, or allow it to settle for a few hours and then decant to a clean bottle, discarding any residue that has gathered at the bottom of the container. Herb Oil will keep for about 1 week in the refrigerator or 1 month in the freezer.

Combining the herbs in a single infusion creates a complex layering of flavors and special effects. The chives bring a mild onion taste to the mix, the watercress adds a peppery tang, and the tarragon pulls the whole thing in an elegant direction. All in all, the result is a highly versatile herb oil that works in a wide spectrum of applications.

Roasted Pepper Oil

Makes about 1¼ cups

2 red bell peppers, roasted (see note)
½ teaspoon sea salt
1 cup Udo's Oil

*P*lace the peppers in a blender with the salt and process on high speed until smooth. Add the oil and blend for about 1 minute longer. Pour the mixture into a glass container, cover, and refrigerate for 8 to 12 hours. Strain through several layers of cheesecloth and return to the refrigerator.

Use the oil as is, or allow it to settle for a few hours and then decant to a clean bottle, discarding any residue that has gathered at the bottom of the container. Roasted Pepper Oil will keep for about 1 week in the refrigerator or 1 month in the freezer.

You'll probably find dozens of applications for this delicious oil, so you may want to double the recipe. Combine it with garlic and hot red chiles for an extra kick. Since the roasting process tends to dehydrate the bell peppers, look for ones with thick flesh, sometimes called Holland or hothouse peppers.

How to Roast Peppers

Preheat the broiler on the highest setting. Quarter the peppers lengthwise and trim away the stem, membranes, and seeds. Arrange the peppers on a baking sheet, skin side up, and roast under the broiler until the skins are blackened. Transfer the peppers to a bowl and cover tightly with a pot lid or foil. Let them steam in their own heat for at least 15 minutes, or until completely cooled. The skins should slip off easily, but if necessary, pry them loose with your fingers and rinse off any blackened bits under running water.

Rosemary Oil

Makes about 1 cup

> 1 cup fresh rosemary leaves (with tender stems only), packed
> 1 cup Udo's Oil
> ½ teaspoon sea salt

Blanch the rosemary in boiling water for about 15 seconds, drain, and immediately plunge into ice water to stop the cooking completely. Chop coarsely and squeeze out the excess water. Combine in a blender with the oil and salt and process for 2 to 3 minutes, until smooth and green. Refrigerate for 8 to 12 hours. Strain through several layers of cheesecloth and return to the refrigerator.

Use the oil as is, or allow it to settle for a few hours and then decant to a clean bottle, discarding any residue that has gathered at the bottom of the container. Rosemary Oil will keep for about 1 week in the refrigerator or 1 month in the freezer.

This is a natural for potatoes and anything bland. It's also good with garlic added and used as a dip or spread for bread.

Scallion Oil

Makes about 1¼ cups

4 cups sliced scallions (white and green parts)
1 cup Udo's Oil
½ teaspoon sea salt

Blanch the scallions in boiling water for 15 seconds, drain, and immediately plunge into ice water to stop the cooking completely. Squeeze out the excess water. Combine the scallions in a blender with the oil and salt and process for 2 to 3 minutes, until bright green. Refrigerate for 8 to 12 hours. Strain through several layers of cheesecloth and return to the refrigerator.

Use the oil as is, or allow it to settle for a few hours and then decant to a clean bottle, discarding any residue that has gathered at the bottom of the container. Scallion Oil will keep for about 1 week in the refrigerator or 1 month in the freezer.

You can actually use this right out of the blender as a strongly flavored purée to garnish soups or other dishes. The portion you don't use right away can then be strained and decanted as directed in the recipe.

SAUCES

They say that variety is the spice of life. If that's true, then the more sauces you know how to make, the spicier your life will be. Sauces also are a terrific way to load essential fatty acids into your diet, because if you manage to make them taste good, you'll eat them as often and as plentifully as you can. In the old days, when people had no refrigeration, sauces masked the taste of rotting meat and fish, making them palatable. (Why didn't they just eat vegetables?) In this glorious day and age of refrigeration and rapid transit, sauces are more of a way to celebrate taste than to cover it up. Are we lucky or what?

The sauces in this book are either Udo-mutated versions of classics or inventions of mine, which means that once you get a feel for how they work, you'll be able to adapt your own favorite recipes to incorporate Udo's Oil into them.

Roasted Red Pepper Sauce

Makes about 2 cups

4 red bell peppers, roasted (see note, page 26)
4 cloves garlic, peeled
$\frac{1}{2}$ teaspoon sea salt
$\frac{1}{2}$ teaspoon cayenne (optional)
$\frac{1}{4}$ teaspoon freshly ground black pepper
$\frac{1}{3}$ cup Udo's Oil

Put the bell peppers, garlic, salt, optional cayenne, and black pepper into a blender and process until smooth. Stir in the oil. Stored in a covered glass container in the refrigerator, Roasted Red Pepper Sauce will keep for up to 2 weeks.

If you plan to make this ahead and will need to heat it, add the oil only after removing the sauce from the heat.

You'll find this a very useful and versatile sauce to have around. Even a small amount in a soup can alter the taste significantly. It stands well on its own, but added to other sauces, it will pull the flavor in a distinct red pepper direction, enriching as it adds an exotic twist. Note that the oil is added at the end, to protect the fragile essential fats.

Chipotle Chili Sauce

Makes about 3 cups

8 Roma tomatoes, coarsely chopped
1 large white onion, coarsely chopped
1 can (7 ounces) chipotle chiles en adobo
7 cloves garlic, peeled
½ teaspoon sea salt
1 to 2 cups vegetable broth
⅓ cup Udo's Oil

*C*ombine the tomatoes, onion, chiles en adobo, garlic, and salt in a blender and process until very smooth, adding a small amount of the broth, if needed. Pour into a saucepan and bring to a simmer. Cook, stirring often, for about 10 minutes, or until the mixture is reduced to a very thick paste. Stir in enough of the broth to create a saucy consistency and simmer for about 10 minutes. Taste and add more salt, if needed. Remove from the heat and stir in the oil, mixing well.

If you don't plan to serve all of the sauce at once, divide it and add the proportion of oil only to the part you are serving. Store the unused portion of sauce in the refrigerator. After you reheat the remaining portion of sauce, add the remaining oil. This way, you won't be heating the oil.

You'll find dozens of applications for Chipotle Chili Sauce. Keep a jar of it in the refrigerator to use on eggs, season beans, or stir into soups—it will add a splash of smoky spice to whatever you're eating. It's a quintessential Mexican flavor, ideal for tacos, tamales, and quesadillas.

Italian Garlic-Chili Oil

Makes about 1½ cups

   4 dried red chiles, stems removed
   ½ cup Italian parsley leaves, packed
   7 cloves garlic, peeled
   1 cup Udo's Oil
   ¼ cup extra-virgin olive oil
   ½ teaspoon sea salt

Put the chiles in a small bowl and cover them with boiling water. Allow them to soften for about 10 minutes.

Wash the parsley in cold water and drain. Press it in a double thickness of paper towels to squeeze out the excess water.

Remove the chiles from the hot water and pat dry. Chop them coarsely with a very sharp knife. Add the garlic and continue chopping until both the chiles and garlic are chopped fairly fine. Add the parsley and continue chopping until everything is finely minced.

Transfer to a small bowl, add the Udo's Oil, olive oil, and salt, and stir well. Taste and add more salt, if needed. Cover until ready to use.

Known to Italians as aglio-olio-peperoncino, this is a sublime sauce for pasta, even whole wheat pasta. It also goes very well with steamed vegetables, especially bland ones such as cauliflower or potatoes, and makes an outstanding dip for bread. If you prefer, you can make this with only Udo's Oil (just replace the olive oil with Udo's Oil) with barely any perceptible difference. Feel free to make this hotter by adding more chiles.

Hoisin Sauce

Makes about 2 cups

1 medium red onion, coarsely chopped
1 cup water
½ cup peeled garlic cloves
½ cup soy sauce
¼ cup honey
¼ cup balsamic vinegar
2 tablespoons Chinese salted black beans (see note)
2 tablespoons tamarind paste (see note)
1 tablespoon Sriracha Sauce (page 38)
1 teaspoon Chinese five-spice powder
1 teaspoon ground licorice root (see note)
2 tablespoons peeled and grated fresh ginger

*P*lace the onion, water, garlic, soy sauce, honey, vinegar, Chinese salted black beans, tamarind paste, Sriracha Sauce, Chinese five-spice powder, and licorice root in a small saucepan and bring to a boil. Adjust the heat to maintain a gentle low simmer, cover, and cook for 15 to 20 minutes, or until the onion and garlic are very tender and the liquid is reduced to a thick syrup. Add a little more water while cooking, if necessary. Remove from the heat and let cool.

Scrape the mixture into a blender, add the ginger, and process until smooth. Stored in a clean glass container in the refrigerator, Hoisin Sauce will keep for at least 1 month.

Chinese salted black beans are one of the most ancient preparations in culinary history. They are boiled, fermented, salted, and aged black soybeans, flavored subtly with ginger. Chinese salted black beans impart a unique flavor to any dish. They should be soft when you buy them. Stored in an airtight container, they will keep indefinitely.

This recipe is provided because it's featured in several other recipes in this book, and because commercial hoisin sauce is an affront to anyone whose health is important to them. (Just read the ingredient panel on the bottle.) This sauce may taste and look slightly different from what is commercially available, but the ingredients are much more healthful.

Tamarind is a tropical tree that produces seed pods containing a dark substance similar to dates with a delicious sweet-sour taste. Used in Asian, African, and Latin American cooking, it is most conveniently found in the form of a paste or concentrate, available in Indian, Middle Eastern, and some specialty shops.

Licorice root is typically a flavor used in European sweets, but in Chinese cooking, it is also used in savory dishes. Both Chinese salted black beans and ground licorice root powder can be found in Asian markets, specialty stores, and some well-stocked supermarkets.

Hollandaise Sauce

Makes about ¾ cup

3 egg yolks
1 tablespoon freshly squeezed lemon juice
¼ teaspoon sea salt
Pinch of cayenne
¼ cup unsalted butter, melted
¼ cup Udo's Oil

*P*lace the egg yolks, lemon juice, salt, and cayenne in a blender and process until well combined. Heat the butter just until it begins to bubble (don't let it brown!). With the blender running, pour in the butter, followed a few seconds later by the oil. The sauce should thicken nicely.

Use at once, or keep the sauce warm for up to 20 minutes by placing it in a bowl set over hot (not boiling) water and whisking it often.

Hollandaise sauce has remained in power, despite all the fad diets that have come and gone, for one reason: it makes everything under it taste like heaven. People are willing (and eager) to continue eating it, even after dire warnings about the attending ills of excessive fat and cholesterol. Here is a minor boon for those who love the taste sensation of hollandaise: half the fat in this recipe is good for you! Unlike butter, essential fats lower cholesterol, improve the absorption of oil-soluble nutrients, and help burn body fat. Now, I don't advocate going hog wild on it, but at least celebrate by having some on your asparagus or broccoli at your earliest convenience. This version of the classic sauce is a bit more fragile than the original, but if you use it right away you should have no problem.

Pesto

2 cups fresh basil leaves, packed
½ cup freshly grated Parmesan cheese
⅓ cup Udo's Oil
2 tablespoons raw pine nuts
4 cloves garlic, peeled
½ teaspoon sea salt
¼ teaspoon freshly ground black pepper
1 tablespoon extra-virgin olive oil

*P*ut the basil, Parmesan cheese, Udo's Oil, pine nuts, garlic, sea salt, and pepper into the work bowl of a food processor and pulse several times to make a uniform paste. This should be done very quickly to avoid heating the ingredients by continued friction. Add a little more oil, if needed, to keep the mixture moving.

When fully blended, scrape into a small container and cover the surface with the olive oil, which will preserve the green color and freshness. Use the sauce immediately, refrigerate it for up to 1 week, or freeze it for up to 3 months.

The traditional Genovese sauce for pasta and gnocchi, pesto's applications are quite diverse. A spoonful added to minestrone or other soups just before serving contributes a delicious enrichment of cheese and a fresh basil flavor. It's good as a sandwich spread, on steamed vegetables or baked potatoes, or stuffed into hollowed-out cherry tomatoes. It's actually fairly addictive, eaten discreetly—or brazenly—directly from a spoon. Stir in the olive oil right before serving, as this will give the pesto just enough authentic olive oil flavor to fool most Italophiles. (Please don't tell them I said this!)

> To avoid heating the ingredients by unnecessary friction, it is helpful to sharpen the blades of the food processor before starting this recipe.

Raw Tomato Sauce

Makes about 3½ cups

- 2 pounds ripe tomatoes
- 1 small onion, very finely diced
- ¼ cup Udo's Oil
- 2 tablespoons extra-virgin olive oil
- 3 cloves garlic, pressed or peeled and minced
- 12 leaves fresh basil, cut into very thin strips
- ½ teaspoon sea salt
- ¼ teaspoon freshly ground black pepper

*C*ut the tomatoes in half crosswise and squeeze gently to extrude the seeds. Dice them finely with a very sharp knife and place them, along with any accumulated juices, in a large glass bowl. Add the remaining ingredients, stir thoroughly, and cover tightly with plastic wrap to keep insects out. Poke several small holes in the plastic with an ice pick. This will release the steam as the mixture marinates, preserving the fresh flavor. Place the bowl outside in the sun for about 1 hour. If you want to capture even more of the sun's rays, spread a sheet of aluminum foil under the bowl, shiny side up.

This is classic summer fare, ideal for alfresco dining—not only eaten outdoors, but prepared outdoors as well. It's an excellent choice anytime you can get good ripe tomatoes, because you'll be able to make tomato sauce without sacrificing the vitamins through cooking. It was intended for spaghetti, and it does that job with distinction, but you'll find many other uses for it, I'm sure. Serve the sauce when it is warm; the aroma will intoxicate anyone within ten feet. Incidentally, it's what has become known as "bruschetta sauce"—which is a complete misnomer, although it does taste good on crostini—so go ahead and use it that way if you want to.

> Tomatoes are rich in lycopene, a powerful antioxidant.

Roasted Garlic Purée

Makes about 2 cups

2 cups peeled garlic cloves
2 tablespoons extra-virgin olive oil
1/2 teaspoon sea salt
1/4 teaspoon freshly ground black pepper
1/2 cup Udo's Oil

Preheat the oven to 375 degrees F. Trim the root ends off the garlic cloves. Toss the garlic in a bowl with the olive oil, salt, and pepper.

Stack 10 sheets of heavy-duty aluminum foil on a work surface and place a sheet of parchment paper on top. Put the garlic mixture in the middle of the paper and fold the parchment and foil over it, crimping the edges to form a tight seal. Place the package in the oven and roast for 45 minutes. Turn the oven down to 325 degrees F and roast for 15 minutes longer. Remove the package from the oven and let cool completely.

Open the package and transfer the roasted garlic and any accumulated juice to a food processor. Add the Udo's Oil and process into a smooth purée. Taste and season with additional salt and pepper, if needed.

Use at once, or scrape into a glass jar or small glass bowl, cover tightly, and refrigerate. Stored in the refrigerator, Roasted Garlic Purée will keep for 2 to 3 weeks.

Garlic becomes quite tame and almost sweet when roasted in this way. There are many applications for this preparation, not the least of which is a dramatic lift for mashed potatoes. You can use it as a sandwich spread (but not before going out on a date) or as an enriching blast of added flavor for sauces, soups, or salad dressings.

Sriracha Sauce

Makes about 2 cups

15 dried red chiles, seeds and stems removed

1 cup water

1/2 cup (4 ounces) palm sugar (see note)

1/2 teaspoon sea salt

1 cup peeled garlic cloves

7 fresh red jalapeño chiles, coarsely chopped

2 tablespoons red wine vinegar

*P*lace the dried red chiles, water, palm sugar, and salt in a small saucepan and bring to a boil. Adjust the heat to maintain a gentle, low simmer, cover, and cook about 15 minutes, or until the chiles are very tender and the liquid has reduced to a syrup. Remove from the heat and add the remaining ingredients. Let the mixture cool slightly.

Transfer to a blender and process until smooth. Pour into a clean glass container. Stored in the refrigerator, Sriracha Sauce will keep for at least 4 weeks.

This sauce is an ingredient in many other recipes in this book. Although it may be more convenient to buy a commercial Sriracha sauce, this could involve an unacceptable compromise, as the ingredients often include refined sugar and preservatives and the bottle is usually plastic. Although this homemade alternative contains no Udo's Oil, it's provided so you can use it in other recipes.

Palm sugar is used extensively in the cuisines of Thailand, Vietnam, Malaysia, and Indonesia. Made from the sap of date or coconut palms, it has a taste and texture similar to brown sugar, but it has a lower glycemic index and is not refined. If you are unable to find it locally, look for mail order sources on the Web. Alternatives are maple sugar, evaporated cane juice granules, Indian *gur*, found at Indian markets, and Mexican *piloncillo*, which is available in Latin markets and some supermarkets.

Salad Dressings

Good news! It's really not hard to make healthful alternatives to those deadly dressings that add gobs of flab to unsuspecting salad eaters who think they're doing themselves a favor by choosing the salad bar over french fries. Of course, as Udo would quickly interject, fried foods are always worse than foods that aren't fried, regardless of what you put on them. But when you consider that the fats in most commercial salad dressings have been attacked with every chemical under the sun, including caustic soda, phosphoric acid, and bleach, and then heated to frying temperatures at some point, you're only slightly better off consuming these fats than the potatoes fried in them. Scary, isn't it?

Back to the good news. In this chapter, you will find plenty of flavorful, easily prepared salad dressings that offer a succulent way to add essential fats to your diet.

For the best results, it would be good to invest in a heavy mortar and pestle, which will make a huge difference to the outcome of a lot of preparations, most notably aïoli. It's also a lot of fun to pound ingredients into a paste, just like humans have for millennia. There's something special about using a tool that has remained unchanged throughout our culinary evolution. However, a food processor is essential for a number of dishes in this book, so if you would need to buy a mortar and pestle but don't want the additional expense at this time, rest assured that you'll get acceptable results with the processor.

Asian Miso Dressing

Makes about ¾ cup

- 4 large cloves garlic, peeled
- 2 tablespoons grated or minced peeled fresh ginger
- 2 tablespoons mellow white miso
- 1 tablespoon honey
- 2 teaspoons Chinese chili-garlic sauce
- 1 teaspoon soy sauce
- 3 tablespoons Udo's Oil
- ¼ cup freshly squeezed lime juice

*P*ound the garlic to a smooth paste in a mortar. Add the ginger, miso, honey, and chili-garlic sauce, pounding as you go. Mash and pound in the soy sauce, then the oil, then stir in the lime juice. Use immediately.

Basil Vinaigrette

Makes about 2 cups

- 1 cup fresh basil leaves, packed
- ½ cup white balsamic vinegar (see note)
- 1 tablespoon Dijon mustard
- 4 cloves garlic, peeled
- 1 teaspoon sea salt
- ½ teaspoon freshly ground black pepper
- 1 cup Udo's Oil

*C*ombine the basil, vinegar, mustard, garlic, salt, and pepper in a blender and process until smooth. With the blender running, slowly pour in the oil. For the best enjoyment, use this dressing immediately.

This recipe, pounded in a mortar, starts out as a paste, which you could use as a sharp condiment served in a small bowl. Then, with the mere addition of lime juice, it becomes a loud salad dressing, perfect for coleslaw. If you don't have a mortar, this would be a good time to get one. But if you would rather not spend the money, don't let that stop you. Go ahead and use a blender, cheapskate. (Just kidding.)

In addition to being a knockout-brilliant salad dressing, this is also (odd as it may sound) good on a baked potato instead of the usual butter, sour cream, and fake bacon bits.

White Balsamic Vinegar

If you absolutely cannot find white balsamic vinegar (which I seriously doubt), try unseasoned rice vinegar. Although this vinaigrette will keep well for several days in the refrigerator, the bright green color may eventually turn to an olive shade because of the acid in the vinegar.

Balsamic Vinaigrette

Makes about 1½ cups

½ cup balsamic vinegar
1 tablespoon Dijon mustard
2 cloves garlic, peeled
1 teaspoon sea salt
½ teaspoon freshly ground black pepper
¾ cup Udo's Oil
¼ cup extra-virgin olive oil

*C*ombine the vinegar, mustard, garlic, salt, and pepper in a blender and process until smooth. With the blender running, slowly pour in the oils. Pour into a clean glass bottle and store in the refrigerator.

For a milder vinaigrette, omit the garlic. If you prefer, omit the olive oil and substitute an equal amount of Udo's Oil.

This is an excellent everyday salad dressing. Work with the proportion of vinegar to oil to achieve an acidity balance that's agreeable to your palate. It keeps for the life of the Udo's Oil (check the expiration date on the bottle), so make a big batch and store it in a dark glass bottle in the refrigerator. That way, you'll always have a delicious salad dressing on hand and no excuse to miss eating salad every day.

Fiery Lemongrass Vinaigrette

Makes about 1½ cups

1 piece (1 inch) peeled fresh ginger, sliced crosswise

2 stalks lemongrass, trimmed and sliced into ½-inch-long pieces

1 green or red chile (Thai or serrano), sliced

½ cup brown rice vinegar

1 cup Udo's Oil

½ teaspoon sea salt

½ teaspoon freshly ground black pepper

*P*ound the ginger, lemongrass, and chile in a mortar with a pestle until pulpy. Transfer to a saucepan and cover with the vinegar. Bring to a gentle simmer, cover, and remove from the heat.

Let steep for about 15 minutes. When completely cool, strain into a bowl and whisk in the oil, salt, and pepper until the mixture emulsifies.

> If the vinaigrette is too acidic, whisk in more oil. If you would like a sharper vinaigrette, add freshly squeezed lime juice to taste.

With a distinct Southeast Asian tang, this is a sharp wake-up for crisp salad greens, watercress, bean sprouts, coleslaw, and bland foods like tofu. This dressing is best used right away, while the aromatics are still bright. However, any leftover dressing will keep fairly well for 1 to 2 days, stored in an airtight jar in the refrigerator.

Fast Greek Salad Dressing

Makes about 1¼ cups

¼ cup Udo's Oil
¼ cup extra-virgin olive oil
¼ cup red wine vinegar
½ teaspoon dry mustard
1 tablespoon chopped fresh oregano, or 1 teaspoon dried
1 or 2 cloves garlic, pressed or peeled and minced
½ teaspoon sea salt
½ teaspoon freshly ground black pepper

Combine all the ingredients in a bowl and whisk thoroughly. Alternatively, combine the ingredients in a jar and shake well. Taste and adjust the seasonings, if needed. Stored in an airtight jar in the refrigerator, Fast Greek Salad Dressing will keep indefinitely.

This recipe uses half Udo's Oil and half olive oil to keep it vaguely authentic. If you don't care, just use straight Udo's Oil. *(Opa!)*

The further back you go in history, the simpler recipes get. A long time ago, people used to just splash a little oil and vinegar on raw vegetables, maybe with a pinch of salt. Even garlic and pepper came later. The Greeks have been eating this way for millennia. Except for the oregano, this is nothing more than a simple oil and vinegar dressing. If you can't find fresh oregano, or don't have time to run out for it, dried oregano works quite well. Relax. It's Greek, not French. *Opa!*

PseUdo French Dressing

Makes about 2 cups

- ½ cup Udo's Oil
- ¼ cup extra-virgin olive oil
- ¼ cup red or white wine vinegar, sherry vinegar, or champagne vinegar
- 1 to 2 teaspoons Dijon mustard
- ¾ teaspoon sea salt
- ½ teaspoon freshly ground black pepper

Combine all the ingredients in a bowl and whisk until emulsified. Alternatively, place the ingredients in a cruet and shake well. *Voila!*

Store any unused dressing in an airtight glass jar or cruet, refrigerated, for up to 2 weeks.

That reddish, so-called French dressing found in supermarkets and salad bars is pure American blasphemy. It exists nowhere in France, and in my opinion, has no valid reason to exist anywhere else either. Unlike Italian dressing, which at least bears a vague resemblance to what Italians put on their salads, French dressing has no recognizable genealogical roots. In France, the favored dressing for everyday salads is simply *vinaigrette*, which serves as a base to which other ingredients are sometimes added to create different types of dressings, such as Roquefort. Herbs are sometimes added or the quantity of mustard is increased, depending on the application, without changing the generic name of "vinaigrette." What this means is that you can do whatever you like with this basic formula, and virtually any variation could be called French dressing. So there. *Au revoir*, red goop!

Quick Ginger Vinaigrette

Makes about ⅓ cup

1 piece (2 inches) peeled fresh ginger, grated
¼ cup Udo's Oil
1 tablespoon balsamic vinegar
¼ teaspoon sea salt
¼ teaspoon coarsely ground black pepper

Squeeze the juice from the grated ginger into a small bowl and discard the pulp. Add the remaining ingredients and whisk furiously until emulsified.

When you want a fast, gingery something to throw on a salad, this is great. If you want it spicy, simply stir in some Sriracha Sauce (page 38). Use this vinaigrette as soon as you've made it for the best flavor.

Because this recipe makes such a small quantity, whisking by hand is the easiest method for preparing it. If you prefer, you can make it in a blender. Instead of grating the ginger, simply slice it crosswise as thinly as possible. Then put it into the blender with the remaining ingredients and process until smooth.

Pu-erh Tea Vinaigrette

Makes about 1 cup

¼ cup unseasoned rice vinegar

1½ tablespoons pu-erh tea leaves

4½ tablespoons Udo's Oil

2 tablespoons honey

2 tablespoons finely diced shallots

½ teaspoon sea salt

¼ teaspoon freshly ground black pepper

2 teaspoons snipped fresh chervil

2 teaspoons snipped chives

*B*ring the vinegar to a boil in a small pot. Remove from the heat and add the tea, swirling to submerge it. Cover and let steep 10 minutes.

Strain the infusion through a very fine mesh sieve, pressing to extract as much flavor as possible. Add the oil, honey, shallots, salt, and pepper and whisk well. Add the chervil and chives and whisk again briefly. For the best results, use this dressing immediately.

Pu-erh is a wonderfully unique tea made from the fermented leaves of a specific broadleaf tea plant found only in a small region in southwestern China. The origin, development, and production of pu-erh tea date back 1,700 years. It's truly delicious. A friend gave me a dime-bag sample of this tea for my birthday once, and I've been a pu-erhoholic ever since. For this vinaigrette, the tea is steeped in rice vinegar, providing an unusual background taste. A little honey is added, permitting the addition of more vinegar without having to add so much oil that the tea flavor is drowned out. Don't worry if you can't get good chervil; omit it and just go ahead with everything else. Imagine this dressing on very subtle-tasting ingredients like buttery greens and yellow tomatoes. This is good, trust me.

Raspberry Vinaigrette

Makes about 2½ cups

  ½ cup raspberry vinegar
  ¼ cup strained raspberry purée
  2 teaspoons dry mustard
  1 teaspoon sea salt
  ½ teaspoon freshly ground black pepper
  1¼ cups Udo's Oil
  ¼ cup extra-virgin olive oil
  1 tablespoon snipped chives
  2 teaspoons finely chopped shallots

Whisk together the vinegar, raspberry purée, mustard, salt, and pepper in a medium bowl. Whisking constantly, slowly add the Udo's Oil and olive oil in a thin stream. Continue whisking until the mixture has emulsified. Stir in the chives and shallots. Raspberry Vinaigrette will keep quite well for up to 2 weeks, stored in an airtight glass jar in the refrigerator.

Raspberry vinegar became popular in the 1980s, during the yuppie feeding frenzy and all the fou-fou nouvelle stuff that fed it. The addition of raspberry purée gives the dressing extra body as well as a note of fresh fruit. Try it with bitter greens, such as Belgian endive, radicchio, or Treviso, or on asparagus spears, blanched tender-crisp.

Roasted Garlic Vinaigrette

Makes about 2½ cups

1 cup peeled garlic cloves

2 tablespoons extra-virgin olive oil

½ teaspoon sea salt

¼ teaspoon freshly ground black pepper

½ cup red wine vinegar (preferably Cabernet or Zinfandel)

3 tablespoons Dijon mustard

1 cup Udo's Oil

Roasting the garlic not only tames the bite, it adds a nice smoky flavor. As Udo would surely mention, be careful to cut away and discard any bits that may have burned during the roasting process. Sad, yes, but by their noble sacrifice, these bits impart a delectable aroma!

Preheat the oven to 375 degrees F. Toss the garlic with the olive oil, salt, and pepper.

Stack 10 sheets of heavy-duty aluminum foil on a work surface and place a sheet of parchment paper on top. Put the garlic mixture in the middle of the paper and fold the parchment and foil over it, crimping the edges to form a tight seal. Place the package in the oven and roast for about 45 minutes. Remove the package from the oven and let cool completely before opening.

Transfer the roasted garlic to a blender along with any accumulated juices in the package. Add the vinegar and mustard and process until smooth. With the blender running, slowly pour in the Udo's Oil. Taste and adjust the seasonings, if needed. Roasted Garlic Vinaigrette will keep for up to 2 weeks, stored in an airtight glass jar in the refrigerator.

Roasted Pepper Vinaigrette

Makes about 2¼ cups

2 red bell peppers, roasted (see note, page 26)
2 cloves garlic, peeled
½ teaspoon sea salt
¼ teaspoon cayenne
¼ teaspoon freshly ground black pepper
½ cup red wine vinegar (preferably Cabernet or Zinfandel)
1 cup Udo's Oil

Put the peppers, garlic, salt, caynenne, and pepper into a blender and process until thoroughly combined. Add the vinegar and process until smooth. With the blender running, slowly pour in the oil. Taste and adjust the seasonings, if needed. Roasted Pepper Vinaigrette will keep for up to 2 weeks, stored in an airtight glass jar in the refrigerator.

The taste of roasted peppers can be rather addictive. Even the smell of peppers roasting is intoxicating. This dressing can double as a cold sauce for steamed or blanched vegetables. Work with the cayenne to achieve the right amount of heat for your taste and the application you have in mind. As a variation, try making this with green or yellow bell peppers—the green with a little chopped green chile and the yellow with no chile at all, or perhaps with a little saffron powder instead.

Tarragon Vinaigrette

Makes about 1⅔ cups

- ¼ cup white balsamic vinegar (see note, page 40)
- 3 tablespoons tarragon Dijon mustard
- 2 tablespoons freshly squeezed lemon juice
- 1 clove garlic, peeled
- ½ teaspoon sea salt
- ½ teaspoon freshly ground black pepper
- ⅔ cup Udo's Oil

*C*ombine the vinegar, mustard, lemon juice, garlic, salt, and pepper in a blender and process until smooth. With the motor running, slowly pour in the oil until the dressing is emulsified.

This is terrific on a salad of green flageolet beans or on sliced tomatoes. If you can't find tarragon mustard, simply substitute with Dijon mustard and add a tablespoon or two of chopped fresh tarragon along with it. Use this vinaigrette as soon as possible after making it. The color will turn an unappetizing muddy olive if it sits too long.

Roasted Garlic–Miso Dressing

Makes about 2 cups

- ¾ cup Udo's Oil
- ½ cup freshly squeezed lemon juice
- ¼ cup Roasted Garlic Purée (page 37)
- ¼ cup mellow white miso
- ¼ cup honey
- ½ teaspoon freshly ground black pepper

*P*lace all the ingredients in a bowl and whisk until thoroughly combined. Taste and add more pepper, if needed. Roasted Garlic–Miso Dressing will keep for up to 2 weeks, stored in an airtight glass jar in the refrigerator.

This is a good choice for chopped salads, which consist mostly of diced vegetables and are suited to assertive, creamy dressings. It's also delicious with mixed field greens, crisp romaine, and iceberg lettuce.

Sesame Dressing

Makes about 2¼ cups

- ½ cup brown rice vinegar
- ½ cup grated carrot
- ½ cup grated daikon
- ½ large sweet onion (such as Maui or Vidalia), chopped (about ½ cup)
- ½ cup raw sesame seeds
- ¼ cup Udo's Oil
- ¼ cup water
- 2 tablespoons soy sauce
- 4 cloves garlic, peeled
- 1 teaspoon sea salt

Place all the ingredients in a blender and process until thoroughly combined. Sesame dressing should be used the day it is made, preferably right away. It will keep for 2 to 3 days, stored in an airtight glass jar in the refrigerator, but the vibrant flavor of the freshly ground vegetables will be lost.

> Typically, this dressing is fairly thick with a slightly chunky texture, so don't be concerned about getting it perfectly blended. As long as it's smooth enough to pour, it'll work just fine.

This is a pseUdo- Japanese salad dressing. Typically, Japanese dressings don't include any oil, but in this one it's barely noticeable, so we can include essential fatty acids without compromising on taste (and with minimal loss of authenticity). It's good on salads with lots of radishes and sprouts. And it's so easy to make—just put everything in a blender and blast away. *Banzai!*

Shiitake-Miso Dressing

Makes about 2¾ cups

¾ ounce dried shiitake mushrooms

5 tablespoons brown rice vinegar

2½ tablespoons soy sauce

2 tablespoons mellow white miso

1 tablespoon raw sesame seeds

1 tablespoon chopped shallots

1 teaspoon minced garlic

1 teaspoon peeled and grated fresh ginger

1 cup plus 2 tablespoons Udo's Oil

Marvelously earthy and exotic tasting, this dressing is good on a wide array of salads, notably any containing Asian greens and sprouts. Consider adding a tablespoon of whole sesame seeds just before serving, along with some thinly sliced scallions. Or, if you prefer, omit the diced shiitakes at the end for an unobstructed, velvety-smooth dressing.

*P*lace the shiitake mushrooms in a small bowl and cover with warm water. Let them soak for at least 20 minutes, until fully reconstituted. Remove the mushrooms from the water, squeezing gently to extract the excess liquid. Reserve the mushroom soaking liquid! Choose one-third of the mushrooms (the best-looking ones) and set aside. Place the remaining mushrooms into a blender along with the vinegar, soy sauce, miso, sesame seeds, shallots, garlic, and ginger. Add 10 tablespoons of the reserved mushroom soaking liquid and process until smooth. With the motor running, slowly add the oil. Pour into a glass jar.

Stack the reserved mushrooms and slice them finely. Turn the slices 90 degrees and cut across the slices to form perfect, tiny dice. Add these to the dressing, cover the jar, and shake. Shiitake–Miso Dressing will keep for up to 2 weeks, stored in an airtight glass jar in the refrigerator.

Spicy Ginger Vinaigrette

Makes about 1⅓ cups

1 cup Udo's Oil

1 piece (2 inches) peeled fresh ginger, thinly sliced crosswise

2 tablespoons freshly squeezed lime juice

1 tablespoon Sriracha Sauce (page 38)

1 tablespoon brown rice vinegar

1 tablespoon hot water

½ teaspoon sea salt

½ teaspoon freshly ground black pepper

Combine all the ingredients in a blender and process until smooth. Taste and adjust the seasonings, if needed. Pour into a glass jar or cruet and let stand at room temperature for at least 1 hour to allow the flavors to develop. Shake well before serving.

> If you're making the vinaigrette a few hours in advance, keep it refrigerated, but bring it to room temperature and shake well before serving. It will keep for up to 1 week, stored in an airtight glass jar in the refrigerator.

This is excellent on crisp salad greens, steamed vegetables, and tofu. If you like the ginger but don't want it spicy, simply omit the Sriracha Sauce.

Sweet Balsamic Vinaigrette

Makes about 1⅓ cups

¼ cup freshly squeezed lemon or lime juice

1½ tablespoons Dijon mustard

7 cloves garlic, peeled

2 tablespoons aged balsamic vinegar (see note, page 111)

2 tablespoons maple syrup

½ teaspoon sea salt

½ teaspoon freshly ground black pepper

⅔ cup Udo's Oil

*P*lace the lemon juice, mustard, garlic, vinegar, maple syrup, salt, and pepper in a blender and process until well combined. With the motor running, slowly pour in the oil until the dressing is emulsified. Sweet Balsamic Vinaigrette will keep for up to 1 week, stored in an airtight glass jar in the refrigerator.

The key to this recipe is using genuine, aged balsamic vinegar. It's expensive, but a little goes a long way. If you don't want to spend the money, you can turn this in the direction of a honey-mustard dressing by using a standard supermarket balsamic, increasing the mustard, and substituting honey for the maple syrup.

DIPS AND CONDIMENTS

Let's face it, unless you're an unusually gung-ho enthusiast, you probably won't be cooking from this cookbook every day. So, in order to keep a steady intake of essential fatty acids flowing seamlessly throughout the week, I suggest preparing some of the dips and condiments in this section whenever you have the time and inclination. These, along with oil infusions, sauces, and salad dressings, may end up being the chief delivery system for adding EFAs to your regular meals, whether they consist of raw or cooked foods served hot, cold, or at room temperature. Having a variety of these at your disposal will enable you to keep essential fats in your diet without a second thought. In addition, you'll be able to entertain friends, treating them to interesting snacks while adhering to your own health regimen. They too will benefit, whether you tell them what's in the food or not. (Aw, go ahead—tell them!)

Whipped Udo-Butter

Makes about 1 cup

4 ounces (1 stick) unsalted butter, softened at room temperature
½ cup Udo's Oil

Whisk the butter until it is very smooth and creamy. Slowly add the oil, little by little, incorporating it thoroughly. Whisk a little longer, making sure the mixture is perfectly smooth. Scrape into a glass container with a tight-fitting lid and refrigerate. Stored in the refrigerator, Whipped Udo-Butter will keep at least 2 weeks, although once you start using it, don't expect it to last that long.

Udo's Choice Mayonnaise

Makes about 1½ cups

¼ cup freshly squeezed lemon juice, strained
1 egg
1 egg yolk
2 teaspoons Dijon mustard
¾ cup almond oil (see note, page 24)
½ cup Udo's Oil

Combine the lemon juice, egg, egg yolk, and mustard in a blender and process until smooth. With the blender running, slowly pour in the almond oil and Udo's Oil in a very thin stream.

Scrape into a jar and refrigerate. Stored in the refrigerator, Udo's Choice Mayonnaise will keep for up to 1 week.

If, like many people, you're addicted to butter, this is a more healthful alternative for using on your hot cereal, bread, and baked potatoes. It has a soft, spreadable consistency, right out of the refrigerator. I wouldn't recommend going hog wild with it (it's still 50 percent butter), but if you're determined to continue using butter for some things, you're a lot better off with this mixture than margarine (which is 100 percent pure evil). For the best flavor, I recommend using European-style cultured butter for this recipe. Actually, I recommend it for every butter application, but in this instance it greatly improves the overall taste, giving it that *je ne sais quoi* cheesy edge.

Mayonnaise is one of the crowned heads of the condiment world. Made properly, it's worth eating; made with Udo's Oil, it's actually good for you! So get rid of all that store-bought garbage. This is so good, so quick, and so easy to prepare, you'll wonder why you ever used anything else. Before you protest this notion, remember that the oil in commercial products is poisonous (fats that kill), while Udo's Oil is health-enhancing (fats that heal). Do the math.

Artichoke Mayonnaise

Makes about 2 cups

  4 large globe artichokes
  ¼ cup freshly squeezed lemon juice
  1 egg yolk
  2 teaspoons Dijon mustard
  ¼ cup Udo's Oil
  ¼ cup almond oil (see note, page 24)

Snip off the sharp tips of the artichoke leaves with scissors. Steam the artichokes until very tender, about 45 minutes. Gently pull off the leaves and gather them in a bowl or on a plate. Cover them and set aside, or place them in the refrigerator for later use.

Remove the hairy choke from the artichoke bottoms. Chop the artichokes coarsely, put them in a blender with the lemon juice, egg yolk, and mustard, and process until smooth. With the blender running, slowly pour in the Udo's Oil and almond oil in a very thin stream.

Scrape into a jar and refrigerate. Stored in the refrigerator, Artichoke Mayonnaise will keep for up to 5 days. Serve it as an appetizer or hors d'oeuvre in a small bowl surrounded by the artichoke leaves for dipping.

As you might have guessed, this recipe is an alternative to melted butter for dipping artichoke leaves. But imagine it as a spread on an open-faced sandwich with stewed leeks and shaved white truffles, for example, or as a base for an unusual salad dressing. Tantalizing, isn't it?

Basil Mayonnaise

Makes about 2¼ cups

¼ cup freshly squeezed lemon juice, strained
1 egg
1 egg yolk
2 teaspoons Dijon mustard
1 cup coarsely chopped fresh basil leaves, packed
¾ cup almond oil (see note, page 24)
½ cup Udo's Oil

Combine the lemon juice, egg, egg yolk, and mustard in a blender and process until smooth. Add the basil and blend thoroughly, stopping to scrape down the sides of the blender jar as needed. With the blender running, slowly pour in the almond oil and Udo's Oil in a very thin stream.

Scrape into a jar and refrigerate. Stored in the refrigerator, Basil Mayonnaise will keep for up to 1 week.

Basil is simply a wonderful herb, period. In this mayonnaise, it really shines. You'll find many ways to use this condiment as a counterpoint to other flavors. For simplicity at its finest, try it as a simple sandwich spread under slices of fresh tomato topped with a sprinkling of Celtic salt and freshly ground black pepper.

Chipotle Mayonnaise

Makes about 2 cups

1 can (7 ounces) chipotle chiles en adobo
1 recipe Udo's Choice Mayonnaise (page 56)

Place the chipotle chiles with their sauce in a blender and process very thoroughly until smooth. Strain through a medium-fine mesh sieve, making sure no seeds get through. Pour into a bowl and gently whisk in the mayonnaise.

Scrape into a sterile jar, cover, and refrigerate. Stored in the refrigerator, Chipotle Mayonnaise will keep for several weeks.

This is a dynamite sandwich spread, certainly, but it's also a sparky condiment to serve with anything that needs a lift. Use it as an ingredient in any number of spicy little inventions. It's even an addictive dip for just about anything. So easy to make; so devastatingly good. Not only that—it'll put to rest, once and for all, that vile redneck gossip about vegetarians being a bunch of anemic wimps.

Parsley Aïoli

Makes about ¾ cup

2 tablespoons chopped fresh parsley
1 egg yolk
2 cloves garlic, peeled
1 slice French bread, crusts removed, soaked in milk and squeezed out
½ cup Udo's Oil

Pound the parsley, egg yolk, and garlic in a mortar with a pestle until well mashed. Add the bread and continue pounding. Pour in tiny dribbles of the oil, using the pestle to stir and beat it into the mixture. When all the oil is incorporated, the mixture will be light and should have the consistency of soft mayonnaise. At this point, the aïoli is at its peak of flavor and texture and is best used immediately. If you cannot use it at once, transfer it to a sterile jar and refrigerate. Stored in the refrigerator, Parsley Aïoli will keep for up to 1 week.

This is good on steamed vegetables and is also a tasty sandwich spread. The key to a velvety aïoli is to pound it by hand in a mortar, adding the oil drop by drop. However, don't let the absence of a mortar (or laziness) stop you from trying this recipe. It's really quite delicious as a sauce or a condiment. If you want to make it runny enough to pour, whisk in a bit of vegetable broth. Don't overdo it— it should still be fairly thick.

Olive Paste

Makes about 1¼ cups

1 cup kalamata olive pulp (about 2 cups olives, well rinsed, pitted, and finely chopped)
½ cup Udo's Oil
1 tablespoon finely chopped fresh parsley
1 tablespoon freshly squeezed lemon juice
2 cloves garlic, peeled, chopped, and mashed to a smooth pulp
¼ teaspoon sea salt
¼ teaspoon freshly ground black pepper

Combine all the ingredients in a small bowl and mix thoroughly. Taste and adjust the seasonings, if needed. Olive Paste will keep for 1 week, stored in an airtight glass jar in the refrigerator.

The original form of this is called *olivada* in Italy, where it's made with tiny Ligurian olives, which are virtually indistinguishable from niçoise olives from Provence, but don't say this in front of any Italians. Once you try it, you'll want to have it on hand at all times. If you don't favor dark olives, try the same recipe with green olives (picholine). Both versions are quite good as a room-temperature sauce for pasta.

Tapenade with a Twist

Makes about 1½ cups

1 cup pitted kalamata olives
¼ cup Simple Garlic Oil (page 22)
3 tablespoons capers, rinsed
1½ ounces dark chocolate, melted
2 tablespoons extra-virgin olive oil
1 tablespoon chopped fresh parsley
1 teaspoon finely grated lemon zest
½ teaspoon cayenne
½ teaspoon chopped fresh thyme

Combine all the ingredients in a food processor and pulse until well mixed but still slightly chunky. The mixture should be spreadable and have some texture.

Scrape into a glass bowl and use immediately, or refrigerate until needed. Before serving, bring to room temperature for the best flavor.

I've always favored kalamata olives. They're juicy and tender, and have a delicious sweet-saltiness that keeps me eating them well after I've had my normal olive fix. In this tapenade, the kalamatas are given an extra kick by the rather unorthodox additions of cayenne and just a bit of melted chocolate. Chocolate is good for you. Once you understand this concept, it's only a matter of discovering as many ways to enjoy it as possible. Most people won't even know it's in this dish, but they'll benefit just the same.

Green Tapenade

Makes about 2 cups · *See photo facing page 65*

1 cup pitted Italian or French green olives
½ cup finely chopped fresh parsley
¼ cup capers, rinsed
¼ cup Simple Garlic Oil (page 22)
1 hard-boiled egg, coarsely chopped
1 tablespoon Dijon mustard
¼ teaspoon sea salt
¼ teaspoon freshly ground black pepper

Combine all the ingredients in a food processor and pulse until well mixed but still slightly chunky. The mixture should be spreadable and have some texture.

Scrape into a glass bowl and use immediately, or refrigerate until needed. Stored this way, it will keep for 2 days. Before serving, bring to room temperature for the best flavor.

There are probably as many versions of tapenade as there are cooks in Provence. The term "tapenade" is derived from *tapeno*, the word for caper in the Provençal dialect. Technically, you can call any condiment tapenade as long as it has capers in it, but you're probably safest if there are olives in it too. Here is an alternative to the usual dark olive tapenade; this one is made with green olives. Be sure to use the right olives—picholine, Sicilian, or Tuscan work well, but not American pitted green olives!

Baba Ghanoush

Makes about 4 cups

2 large eggplants
1 cup chopped fresh parsley
1/4 cup freshly squeezed lemon juice
4 cloves garlic, peeled
1 teaspoon sea salt
1 1/2 cups tahini
1/2 cup Udo's Oil
Extra-virgin olive oil
Kalamata olives
Parsley leaves

Grill the whole eggplants, turning them occasionally so all sides are evenly cooked, for 15 to 20 minutes, or until they are tender to the touch. Let cool. Slit open the eggplants, scoop out the flesh (and discard the skins), and place in a food processor along with the chopped parsley, lemon juice, garlic, and salt. Process until well blended. With the motor running, add the tahini, a spoonful at a time, followed by the Udo's Oil. Process until smooth. The mixture will be a light beige color with a beautiful greenish tint from the little flecks of parsley.

Spread in a shallow dish, making a shallow, circular trough in the surface with the back of a spoon. Pour olive oil into the trough and decorate the dish with the olives and parsley leaves.

Sadly, there are very few recipes for eggplant that don't include some form of frying, grilling, or browning, all of which are hostile to one's health, as explained by Udo. Here is one in which the unburned portion of the eggplant is salvaged and used as the incomparable base for a dear favorite of mine. Serve it with pita bread or fresh raw vegetables.

If you enjoy extra garlic, increase the number of cloves to taste. If you would like to prepare this dish in advance, omit the final step of garnishing with olive oil, olives, and parsley; cover the dish tightly with plastic wrap and refrigerate until about 20 minutes before serving time. Remove the Baba Ghanoush from the refrigerator, allow it to come to room temperature, and proceed with the final touches. Leftover Baba Ghanoush will keep several days, tightly covered, in the refrigerator.

Hummus

Makes about 3½ cups

1½ cups cooked chickpeas
½ cup freshly squeezed lemon juice
4 cloves garlic, peeled
1½ teaspoons sea salt
1 cup tahini
¾ cup Udo's Oil
2 tablespoons extra-virgin olive oil
Parsley sprigs

*P*lace the chickpeas in a food processor along with the lemon juice, garlic, and salt and process until smooth. With the processor running, add the tahini, a spoonful at a time, followed by the Udo's Oil. If the mixture becomes too thick, add a little water or more lemon juice. Taste and adjust the flavorings as you see fit.

Spread in a wide, shallow dish, drizzle with the olive oil, and garnish with parsley sprigs.

If you enjoy extra garlic, increase the number of cloves to taste. If you would like to prepare this dish in advance, omit the final step of garnishing with olive oil and parsley; cover the dish tightly with plastic wrap and refrigerate until about 20 minutes before serving time. Remove the Hummus from the refrigerator, allow it to come to room temperature, and proceed with the final touches. Leftover Hummus will keep several days, tightly covered, in the refrigerator.

This might very well be the most popular dip in the world. Versions of hummus are served all over the Middle East, with varying proportions of tahini, garlic, and lemon juice. Feel free to experiment with the quantities until you've got a combination that suits your palate. Most people prefer not to spend a lot of time cooking chickpeas, so don't feel even the slightest hesitation about using canned. Just make sure they're organic and drain them before measuring. Serve this dish with whole wheat pita bread or vegetables for dipping.

Red Pepper and Walnut Dip

Makes about 4½ cups

See photo facing page 65

1½ teaspoons ground cumin

2½ pounds red bell peppers, roasted (see note, page 26)

1½ cups raw walnuts

¼ cup Udo's Choice Wholesome Fast Food (see note, page 65)

¼ cup pomegranate molasses (see note, page 65)

¼ cup Udo's Oil

1 tablespoon freshly squeezed lemon juice

1 teaspoon honey

1 teaspoon cayenne

¾ teaspoon sea salt

2 tablespoons extra-virgin olive oil

1 to 2 tablespoons chopped raw pistachios

5 to 6 cilantro sprigs

*T*oast the cumin in a small skillet until it releases a rich aroma. Immediately remove the skillet from the heat and put the cumin into a food processor along with the peppers, walnuts, Udo's Choice Wholesome Fast Food, pomegranate molasses, Udo's Oil, lemon juice, honey, cayenne, and salt. Process the mixture as smoothly as possible, stopping occasionally to scrape down the sides of the work bowl as needed. Taste and adjust the seasonings, if needed.

recipe continues on next page

This variation of a seriously delectable Middle Eastern classic is excellent with pita bread as well as raw vegetables. To be quite honest, it's downright addictive, so you might want to make a double amount. It keeps well for several days (not that it will last that long).

Photo (clockwise from left): Zucchini Boats with Roasted Garlic Purée (page 88), Fava Bean Purée (page 70) on toasts with shaved Pecorino Pepato Oven-dried Tomatoes with Pesto and Brie (page 85) Asparagus-stuffed Eggs (page 82)

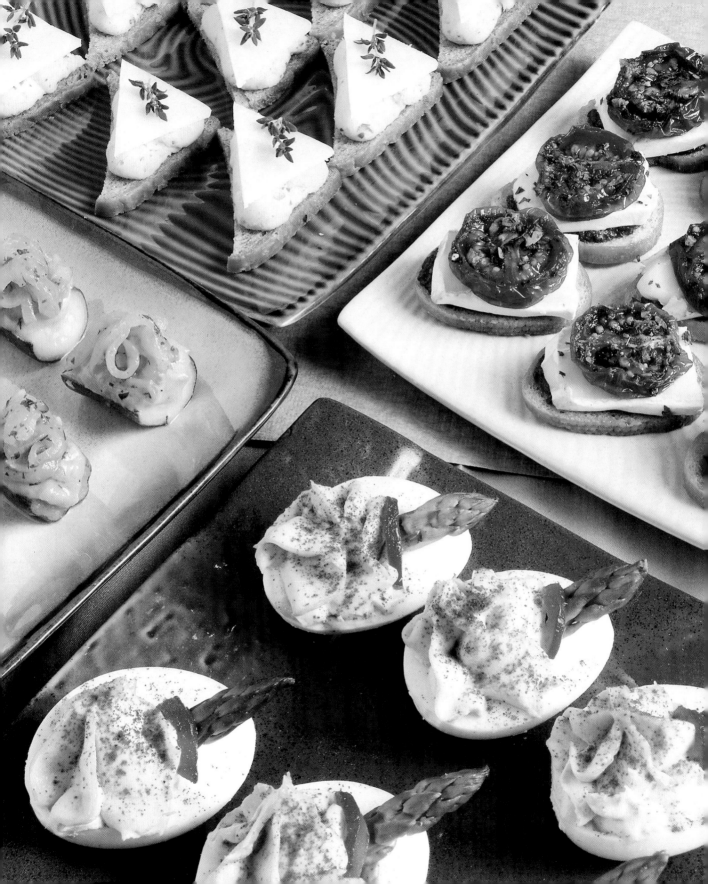

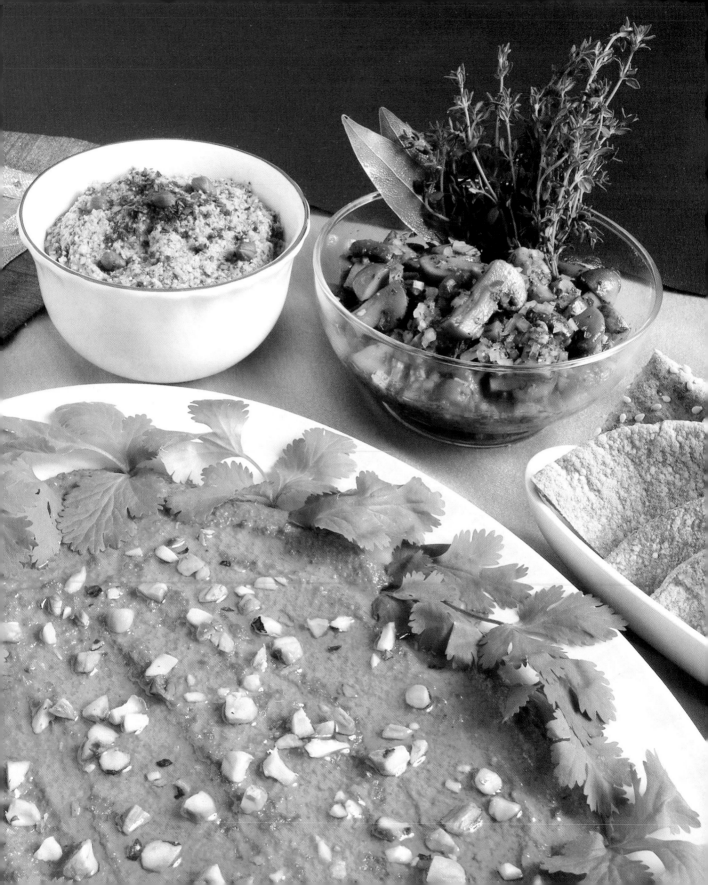

Pour into a wide, shallow serving dish and spread into an even layer. Drizzle the olive oil over the top, sprinkle with the pistachios, and garnish with the cilantro sprigs. Serve at room temperature.

If you would like to prepare this dish in advance, omit the final step of garnishing with olive oil, pistachios, and cilantro sprigs; cover the dish tightly with plastic wrap and refrigerate until about 20 minutes before serving time. Remove the dip from the refrigerator, allow it to come to room temperature, and proceed with the final touches. Leftover Red Pepper and Walnut Dip will keep several days, tightly covered, in the refrigerator.

Pomegranate molasses is a staple in the Middle East. It can be found in Middle Eastern grocery stores and even in many supermarkets. If you can't locate any, you can make your own easily by boiling pomegranate juice until it is reduced to a thick syrup. Pomegranate juice is now widely available in most supermarkets. However, check the ingredients carefully, as these often include other fruit juices; it's important to use pure pomegranate juice for this preparation.

Udo's Choice Wholesome Fast Food is a powdered, nutrient-rich mixture of natural-source fibers with added whole food concentrates, essential fats, phytonutrients, greens, and digestive enzymes. It is designed to deliver optimum nutrition, resulting in increased energy, stable blood sugar, greater bowel regularity, and lower cholesterol. As for it by name at your natural food store.

*Photo: Red Pepper and Walnut Dip (page 64),
Green Tapenade (page 61),
Marinated Mushrooms (page 71)*

Mexi-Hummus

Makes about 3 cups

1½ cups cooked black beans
½ cup fresh cilantro, firmly packed
⅓ cup freshly squeezed lime juice
7 cloves garlic, peeled and coarsely chopped
1 fresh green serrano chile, coarsely chopped
1½ teaspoons sea salt
¾ cup tahini
⅓ cup Udo's Oil
2 tablespoons extra-virgin olive oil
Cilantro sprigs

Place the black beans in a food processor along with the ½ cup cilantro, lime juice, garlic, green chile, and salt and process until smooth. With the processor running, add the tahini, a spoonful at a time, followed by the Udo's Oil. If the mixture becomes too thick, add a little water or more lime juice.

Spread in a wide, shallow dish, drizzle with the olive oil, and garnish with cilantro sprigs.

Okay, so we have a kind of heresy here, mixing cultures like this. So what! Call me an infidel. Try it once. Black beans, cilantro, and green chile give hummus a Mexican flavor, yet the overall effect is not at all un–Middle Eastern. It's spicy, pungent, and addictive. Get out the pita bread!

If you enjoy extra heat, increase the number of chiles to taste. If you would like to prepare this dish in advance, omit the final step of garnishing with olive oil and cilantro sprigs; cover the dish tightly with plastic wrap and refrigerate until about 20 minutes before serving time. Remove the Mexi-Hummus from the refrigerator, allow it to come to room temperature, and proceed with the final touches. Leftover Mexi-Hummus will keep several days, tightly covered, in the refrigerator.

Black Bean Relish

Makes about 3½ cups

1 green bell pepper, roasted (see note, page 26)

1 yellow bell pepper, roasted (see note, page 26)

2 cups cooked black beans

1 firm ripe avocado, diced

1 small red onion, finely diced

8 scallions, thinly sliced

¼ cup Udo's Oil

¼ cup coarsely chopped fresh cilantro

2 tablespoons freshly squeezed lime juice

2 or more serrano chiles, finely diced

4 cloves garlic, peeled and minced

*D*ice the peppers and place them in a glass bowl. Add all the remaining ingredients and stir gently until thoroughly combined. Cover tightly and refrigerate until ready to use. Technically, this dish will keep for a few days in the refrigerator, but most of its vibrant, fresh qualities will be gone by the next morning. Better to eat it all up the day it is made.

An unorthodox but welcome relative of Mexican salsa, this is a great all-around accompaniment for virtually any informal meal, especially one with a Latin American flavor.

Chipotle Chili Paste

Makes about 3½ cups

4 dried chipotle chiles
2 cups hot vegetable broth
2 Roma tomatoes, coarsely chopped
½ medium white onion, coarsely chopped
7 cloves garlic, peeled
½ teaspoon sea salt
1 bay leaf
3 tablespoons Udo's Oil

Put the chipotle chiles in a bowl and pour the hot broth over them. Let them soak for at least 1 hour, until fully reconstituted. Pour the broth and chiles into a blender and add the tomatoes, onion, garlic, and salt. Process until completely smooth, making sure there are no seeds remaining. Strain through a medium-fine mesh sieve, pour into a saucepan, add the bay leaf, and bring to a simmer. Cook until the mixture is greatly reduced, very thick, and almost dry. As the mixture thickens, stir often. Remove from the heat, remove and discard the bay leaf, and whisk in the oil.

Transfer to an airtight glass container and store in the refrigerator for up to 3 weeks.

I find this utterly indispensable, as I can quickly make other things with it, such as Chipotle Mayonnaise (page 58), or add it to various dishes to spice them up. Although you can get basically the same result by simply blending a can of chipotles en adobo, this is a way to make chili paste from scratch, using only the most health-promoting ingredients. Use it sparingly, as it is very spicy!

Corn Relish

2 cups fresh corn kernels

1 red bell pepper, roasted (see note, page 26) and diced

1 small red onion, finely diced

8 scallions, thinly sliced

2 tablespoons Udo's Oil

2 tablespoons coarsely chopped fresh cilantro

1 tablespoon brown rice vinegar

4 cloves garlic, peeled and minced

1 teaspoon hot chili and garlic paste (see note)

*B*lanch the corn in boiling salted water for 2 minutes. Drain and immediately plunge in ice water to stop the cooking completely. Drain thoroughly and transfer to a glass bowl. Add all of the remaining ingredients and mix well. Cover tightly and refrigerate until ready to use. Technically, this dish will keep for a few days in the refrigerator, but most of its vibrant, fresh qualities will be gone by the next morning. Better to eat it all up the day it is made.

This is a kind of fusion-cuisine thing, combining Latin American ingredients with Indonesian chili paste. Unlike a lot of the anything-goes mishmash nonsense you run into these days, this one works. It rocks, actually.

Sambal Oelek

Hot chili and garlic paste is also known as Indonesian *sambal oelek*. It is available in Asian grocery stores and in many supermarkets in the Asian section. If you can't locate sambal oelek, make your own by mashing garlic and crushed red chiles with a little salt and oil. It's not rocket science—just wing it!

Fava Bean Purée

Makes about 2¼ cups   *See photo facing page 64*

2 cups shelled fresh fava beans (about 5 pounds unshelled)
2 cloves garlic, peeled, mashed, and minced
¾ teaspoon sea salt
½ teaspoon freshly ground black pepper
½ cup Udo's Oil

*B*lanch the fava beans in lightly salted water for about 3 minutes. Drain, refresh under cold water, and drain again. Pinch the skins on the indented side and slip out the beans. (Take a minute to marvel at the striking beauty of these gorgeous green little things.) If you have a mortar and pestle, pound the beans into a paste along with the garlic, salt, and pepper. When the paste is smooth, begin adding the oil, 1 teaspoon at a time, pounding and churning as you go. Once all the oil is incorporated, scrape the purée into a bowl and cover tightly until ready to serve, up to 1 hour. To keep longer, refrigerate and then let it come to room temperature before serving. Tightly covered, it will keep in the refrigerator for 2 to 3 days.

If you don't have a mortar and pestle, use a food processor, following the same procedure. The result will be nearly the same, only a bit less silky.

This is a good spread for little hors d'oeuvre items, but it stands well on its own on a plate with most entrées. Try not to think about Hannibal Lecter, although a good Chianti does wash it down rather nicely.

Marinated Mushrooms

Makes about 2 cups

See photo facing page 65

1 pound small cremini mushrooms

1 teaspoon minced garlic

1 teaspoon sea salt

½ teaspoon freshly ground black pepper

1 bay leaf

¼ cup water

½ cup Udo's Oil

2 tablespoons finely chopped shallots

1 tablespoon chopped fresh thyme, or 1 teaspoon dried

*W*ash the mushrooms well and trim the stems to about ¼ inch. Place in a saucepan with the garlic, salt, pepper, bay leaf, and dried thyme, if using. Add the water, cover, and bring to a simmer over high heat. Remove the lid and cook until the mushrooms are tender and only a few tablespoons of liquid remain. Remove from the heat and stir in the oil, shallots, and fresh thyme, if using. Let cool completely. Serve at room temperature or refrigerate and serve cold. Stored in a glass jar or bowl, tightly covered and refrigerated, Marinated Mushrooms will keep for 1 week with impunity.

Marinated mushrooms are a standard member of the antipasto family, including traditional Italian antipasto and all of its relatives found throughout the Mediterranean countries. It's a good snack, too, for insomniacs rifling through the refrigerator in the middle of the night.

Oily Salsa

See photo facing page 128

Makes about 4¾ cups

4 to 6 plump Roma tomatoes, finely diced (about 3 cups)

1 medium white onion, finely diced (about 1 cup)

½ cup coarsely chopped fresh cilantro

¼ cup Udo's Oil

4 or more green serrano chiles, finely diced

2 to 3 tablespoons freshly squeezed lime juice

1 or 2 cloves garlic, peeled and minced

¾ teaspoon sea salt

*C*ombine all the ingredients in a glass bowl and stir until thoroughly combined. If time permits, let rest at room temperature for at least 15 minutes to allow the flavors to develop. Stir again and serve.

The word "salsa" is widely used and rarely understood, even when it's obvious that the context is food and not music. All the word means is "sauce." So no one should be shocked or flipped out if we add oil to the Mexican fresh condiment most commonly referred to as "salsa." I think most Mexicans would be quite accepting of any sauce that sets their mouths on fire. So here we go!

This salsa should really be used the day it is made for the best flavor. However, it can be stored in the refrigerator for up to 3 days. Even though the taste may suffer a bit, it will still be a great condiment.

Harissa

Makes about 2 cups

3 red bell peppers, roasted (see note, page 26)

6 to 8 fresh red jalapeño chiles, coarsely chopped (see note)

2 cloves garlic, peeled

1 teaspoon lightly toasted caraway seeds

½ teaspoon sea salt

6 tablespoons Udo's Oil

*P*lace the peppers in a blender along with the chiles, garlic, caraway seeds, and salt. Process into a smooth paste. With the blender running, add the oil and process until well mixed. Taste and adjust the seasonings, if needed. Scrape into a glass jar and store in the refrigerator for up to 2 weeks.

Harissa is a very spicy North African condiment for vegetables, soups, and stews. The one ingredient that makes it uniquely Moroccan isn't the peppers but the caraway seeds. A dab of this in an otherwise pedestrian soup will immediately transform it into something spectacular.

If you are unable to find any fresh red jalapeños, substitute 1 to 2 tablespoons crushed dried red chiles.

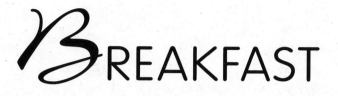

BREAKFAST

I grew up in Mexico, where we always ate a huge breakfast right after dawn. Then I went to Europe, where most people start the day with a stout cup of coffee and some form of bread, and then have a substantial snack around midmorning. While I found this infinitely more civilized, it did tend to put me out of sync with the normal schedule when I eventually ended up in the United States. Finally, I've come to a compromise: get up early, eat after being awake at least an hour, and make the morning meal count without overdoing it. Sound reasonable?

Whatever your situation or predilection may dictate regarding the time for your first meal of the day, you'll find a few good options in this section. Traditional Western breakfasts have tended toward either a sweet dish, usually cereal, or some combination of eggs, meat, and potatoes. The challenge inherent in duplicating these sorts of breakfast dishes using healthful (as well as ethical and sustainable) alternatives lies not only in the substitution of ingredients but also in the cooking methods. Hopefully, the following recipes will manage to bridge the acceptability gap.

Sweet Udo

Makes about ⅔ cup

    ¼ cup Udo's Oil
    ¼ cup honey
    2 tablespoons agave nectar (see note) or additional honey
    1 teaspoon crushed cardamom seeds (see note)

*P*ut all of the ingredients in a small bowl and whisk furiously until the mixture is emulsified.

Agave nectar, called *agua miel* in Mexico, is a delicious extract from the agave plant. It was discovered by the Toltecs a few thousand years ago and became a staple in their diet, providing a rich source of minerals. They loved the stuff so much that at one point they decided to stockpile it. Big mistake. Unfortunately, their supply fermented after a period of time, producing a hideous milky liquor (now known as *pulque*), to which they took a particular liking. Native Americans are genetically indisposed to handle alcohol (perhaps to their credit), and the Toltecs were no exception. Their sophisticated culture declined after that, and eventually they were conquered by the invading Chichimecas, an entirely inferior society whose only strength was warfare. Incidentally, tequila is a distilled version of the same stuff. Any questions?

Okay, so your kids probably aren't going to go for the Udo lifestyle in a big way. Here's an excellent middle ground, where you can get some goodness into them while they're not looking. The only compromise is toasting the bread. Be aware that once the mixture is made it should be used right away or it will separate. If you prefer, use cinnamon instead of cardamom.

Cardamom is a wonderfully fragrant Asian spice, used for both sweet and savory dishes. Look for it in Indian and Middle Eastern shops, either in whole green pods or decorticated (removed from the pod). In some Indian dishes, the cardamom pod is added whole, but for most other uses, only the seeds are used; the outer husk is discarded. Always crush cardamom seeds at the time of use, for the best flavor and the most health benefits. In traditional Indian and Chinese medicine, cardamom is used to treat pulmonary congestion, digestive disorders, and infections in the mouth.

Wholesome Applesauce

Makes about 1½ cups

  1 cup applesauce
  ⅓ cup Udo's Oil
  2 to 3 tablespoons Udo's Choice Wholesome Fast Food
    (see note, page 65)
  1 capsule Udo's Choice Enzyme Blend (see note)

*S*coop the applesauce into a bowl. Make a small well in the center and pour the oil into it. Sprinkle the remaining ingredients onto the oil and stir in, slowly incorporating the applesauce until well blended. If the mixture becomes too thick, add a little apple juice or water. Eat!

This isn't my recipe, and I'll admit that when Udo explained it to me, I had serious doubts. But after trying it, I'm a convert. Weird as it may sound, it's a keeper. Don't even think about making this ahead of serving time—it sets up rather quickly, so plan to eat it right away (unless you need something to stick model airplane parts together).

Udo's Choice Enzyme Blend contains a full spectrum of precisely balanced different plant digestive enzymes: amylase, cellulase, glucoamylase, invertase, lactase, lipase, malt diastase, pectinase, phytase, protease, and bromelain.

Apple-Carrot Oat Bran Cereal

Makes 2 servings

2 cups apple juice

2 cups carrot juice

½ teaspoon ground cardamom (see note, page 74)

¼ teaspoon freshly grated nutmeg

⅛ teaspoon sea salt

1½ cups oat bran

1 large carrot, grated

1 apple, grated

Sweet Udo (page 74) or Whipped Udo-Butter (page 56)

Combine the apple juice, carrot juice, cardamom, nutmeg, and salt in a heavy saucepan and bring to a boil. Slowly pour in the oat bran, whisking vigorously to break up any lumps. As soon as the mixture returns to a boil, turn the heat down to the lowest setting and cook, uncovered, whisking often, for about 2 minutes. Stir in the carrot and apple. Cook for about 2 minutes longer. Serve immediately, with Sweet Udo or Whipped Udo-Butter on the side.

Oat bran was all the rage for a while. Cholesterophobics were shoveling it down in every conceivable vehicle, especially the coffee shop muffin, which they slathered with the utterly nonessential fat, butter (go figure), hoping it would save them from heart attacks, strokes, and colon cancer. Fortunately, the fanaticism has abated somewhat (extremes are scary), but for those who have a reasonable interest in the benefits of oat bran, here's one pretty good way to ingest a dose.

Cashew-Blueberry Kefir

Makes about 4½ cups

2 cups raw cashew pieces
1 cup unsweetened shredded dried coconut
4 cups water
12 capsules Udo's Choice Probiotics (see note)
1 cup blueberries
¼ cup Udo's Oil

Soak the cashews and coconut in the water for 8 to 12 hours. Pour into a blender and process until smooth. With the motor running, open the capsules and add the probiotics (discarding the capsules). The blending action will slightly warm and activate the probiotics, which will help thicken the mixture.

Strain the mixture through a medium-fine mesh sieve, pressing down on the solids to express as much liquid as possible into a clean glass container. Keep in a warm place for 12 hours. The mixture should have a slightly sour taste, similar to yogurt.

Return the mixture to the blender, add the blueberries and oil, and process until smooth. Drink the desired amount at once. Cover the remaining kefir and refrigerate it for up to 3 days.

The addition of coconut to this beverage gives it a delicious flavor and pleasing sweetness so that no added sweeteners are needed. You can use other berries if you prefer. Cashew–Blueberry Kefir can be enjoyed on its own, or as a base for smoothies with the addition of your favorite protein powder.

Udo's Choice Probiotics provides beneficial bacteria to support the immune system, helps the body produce various essential prostaglandins for balancing hormones, and helps prevent pathogenic organisms from gaining a foothold in the body. Ask for it by name at your natural food store.

Essene Bread

Makes 1 loaf

2 cups wheat berries
1 teaspoon sea salt

*P*lace the wheat berries in a 1-gallon glass jar and cover with a double layer of cheesecloth, securing it in place with a heavy rubber band. Fill the jar with filtered water and let the wheat berries soak for 12 hours. Leaving the cheesecloth in place to keep the wheat berries contained, drain, rinse with fresh water, and drain again thoroughly. Lay the jar on its side, away from direct sunlight, and leave the wheat berries to sprout, rinsing and draining again in the evening. On the following day, do not rinse.

Preheat the oven to 200 degrees F. Grind the sprouted berries in a food processor to produce a dense, moist mass. Form into a flat, rectangular loaf about 1½ inches high and place on a baking sheet lightly oiled with lecithin or extra-virgin olive oil. Bake for 2½ to 3 hours, or until the loaf offers resistance when pressed lightly.

The original recipe for this bread appears in The Essene Gospel of Peace, in which Jesus gives the people of his time some valuable health tips (who knew he could cook?). The method in the good book calls for baking the bread in the sun on a hot rock. For those of us who do not live in the Middle East or Death Valley, a low oven will work just as well. If, like many people these days, you have a sensitivity to wheat, whole spelt berries can be substituted with perfectly delicious results. This item has no Udo's Oil in it, so of course you'll want to slather every slice you eat with any of the various spreads and condiments in this book.

This bread will not resemble leavened bread. It will have a tender crust and a moist, chewy texture. To cut the loaf, dip a serrated bread knife in water and use a gentle sawing motion. Wrap the unused portion tightly with parchment or waxed paper, and then in aluminum foil (avoid direct contact with the foil to prevent aluminum contamination). Store the bread in the refrigerator for up to 1 week, or freeze for up to 1 month.

Fruity Quinoa Cereal

Makes about 4½ cups

3 cups apple juice

¼ teaspoon sea salt

1 cup quinoa (see note), well rinsed and drained

¼ cup dried apricots, chopped

¼ cup dried blueberries

¼ cup dried papaya, chopped

¼ cup dried cranberries

½ teaspoon ground cinnamon

¼ teaspoon freshly grated nutmeg

Pinch of ground cloves

Pinch of ground allspice

1 ripe peach, cut into ½-inch pieces

Sweet Udo (page 74) or Whipped Udo-Butter (page 56)

*B*ring the juice and salt to a boil in a medium pot. Stir in the quinoa, dried fruits, and spices. As soon as the mixture returns to a boil, turn the heat down to medium and cover the pot. Cook for about 15 minutes. Uncover, stir in the peach pieces, and check the consistency of the cereal. If it's getting a bit thick, add a little more juice. Cover again and cook for about 5 minutes longer. Serve immediately, with Sweet Udo or Whipped Udo-Butter on the side.

This wonderful grain, quinoa, offers interesting flavor, texture, high protein, and many valuable nutrients. It's a terrific way to start the day.

Instead of apple juice, try apple-pear, cherry, blueberry, or any other subacid fruit juice.

If peaches aren't in season, don't worry—it'll still taste great. Just follow the recipe as if the peaches were in there, perhaps adding a bit more juice for the last few minutes of the cooking time to keep the cereal from getting too dry.

Quinoa, referred to as the "mother grain" by the Incas, is a highly nutritious food. It is a complete protein, gluten free, and easily digested. It is high in magnesium and iron, and is a good source of both phosphorus and dietary fiber. Quinoa can be found in natural food stores and well-stocked supermarkets.

Poached Eggs
with Avocado and Chipotle Sauce

Makes 2 servings

See photo facing page 128

2 large avocados

1 lime, cut into quarters

1 teaspoon white vinegar

4 large, very fresh eggs

1½ cups Chipotle Chili Sauce (page 31)

½ cup grated Monterey Jack or Vermont cheddar cheese
(dairy or soy)

1 tablespoon chopped fresh cilantro

Corn tortillas, warmed (see note)

This is an adaptation of the classic Mexican dish *huevos rancheros*. In this version the eggs aren't fried and the tortillas are on the side. You might serve it with Pinto Beans with Scallions and Cilantro (page 148) for a hearty breakfast or brunch.

Cut the avocados in half, remove the pit, and carefully scoop the flesh out of the skin with a large spoon, keeping each half in one piece. Squeeze the lime over the pieces, coating them thoroughly. Trim the round bottom of the avocado halves slightly so they will sit flat on a plate. Place two avocado halves on each plate.

Bring about 3 inches of water to a boil in a deep sauté pan or wide saucepan. Reduce the heat to maintain a very gentle simmer and add the vinegar. Crack the eggs, one at a time, and carefully open them very close to the surface of the water. If the eggs are very fresh, they should hold together in a nice clump. The vinegar acts as an astringent, helping to keep them from spreading out into the water. Use a large spoon to separate them if they get too close together. Poach the eggs for about 4 minutes (if you like the yolk runny). Lift them out with a slotted spoon and let them drain briefly on a towel.

While the eggs are poaching, heat the Chipotle Chili Sauce as directed in the recipe. Place a poached egg on top of each avocado half. Spoon the chili sauce over them and sprinkle with the cheese. Garnish with the cilantro and serve immediately. Pass the tortillas!

Heating Tortillas

The classic way to heat corn tortillas is to lay them directly on the stove grill, over a gas flame, and flip them often to prevent burning. The other way is to do the same thing but in a hot skillet. After each tortilla is heated through, slip it into a folded napkin or towel. Stack the tortillas together to keep them warm and moist.

Hors d'Oeuvres

The beauty of hors d'oeuvres is that you can have them virtually anytime, whether you're hosting an informal gathering with Chardonnay sippers, whetting your guests' appetites before a fine meal, or just watching TV by yourself. Naturally, since they take a little doing, you'll probably want to wait until you have a wide audience, but once you get accustomed to putting them together, it'll become easy enough to do without much fuss. You might find that you like eating this way as much as any other.

There are only a few recipes in this section, but bear in mind that a lot of the items in the other sections, such as Dips and Condiments, serve very well as hors d'oeuvres. The Artichoke Mayonnaise recipe (page 57) includes directions for this purpose. Any of the dips or aïoli presented with an array of raw or lightly blanched vegetables is another quick choice. Belgian endive or small romaine lettuce leaves can be used as vehicles for Fava Bean Purée (page 70) or one of the tapenades, perhaps with a thin slice of Parmesan or pecorino cheese on top. With just a little practice, you'll easily come up with other ways to use the recipes in this book to make succulent little bites for quick snacking or stimulating your guests' appetites before dinner.

You'll need a baking sheet for some of these recipes. I use commercial aluminum pans because they conduct heat well, but I always place a sheet of parchment paper on them to protect the food from metal contamination.

Asparagus-Stuffed Eggs

Makes 12 pieces

See photo facing page 64

1 pound medium asparagus

6 eggs

¼ cup Udo's Choice Mayonnaise (page 56)

2 teaspoons Dijon mustard

1 teaspoon freshly squeezed lemon juice

⅛ to ¼ teaspoon sea salt

½ red bell pepper, roasted (see note, page 26) and cut
    into ¼-inch-thick strips

Paprika

It's deceptively easy to make this chic version of the old standard deviled egg. The only real work is roasting, peeling, and trimming the red peppers. If you want a lazy person's way out, you can buy a jar of sliced pimientos, which work just fine. Drain them well first, of course.

Snap off and discard the tough ends of the asparagus. Wash the asparagus well. Cut off the tips to a length of about 1½ inches. Cut the stems into ½-inch lengths and keep them separate from the tips. Blanch the tips in boiling water until tender-crisp, remove with a slotted spoon, and refresh under cold water. Drain and spread on a towel to dry. Boil the stems until very tender, drain, refresh in cold water, and squeeze firmly in a towel to remove all the water. Don't worry if the stems fall apart when you squeeze them; they should be a pulpy mass. Place the stems in a food processor.

Bring 1 quart of water to a boil. Gently lower the eggs into the water with a slotted spoon. Lower the heat and boil the eggs gently for 10 minutes. Remove the eggs with a slotted spoon and immediately plunge them into ice water. Peel the eggs carefully in order to keep them whole. Cut them in half lengthwise and scoop out the yolks. Add the yolks to the asparagus stems in the food processor along with the mayonnaise, mustard, lemon juice, and salt. Process until smooth.

If the mixture seems a bit too dry, add a little more mayonnaise and process again until it is incorporated.

Scrape the mixture into a pastry bag fitted with a medium to large star tip. Place an asparagus tip on each egg white half, with the tip sticking out of the cavity, facing the narrow end. Pipe the yolk mixture into the cavities, dividing it as equally as possible. Drape a pepper strip over the asparagus tip, right where it emerges from the yolk mixture. Sprinkle with paprika and serve.

If you want to make these in advance, keep them refrigerated until serving time, and wait until just before serving to sprinkle the paprika. Otherwise, the paprika will absorb moisture and become part of the egg mixture (unattractively so) instead of remaining as a garnish. If you must prepare this recipe far in advance, it is also a good idea to add the pepper strips close to serving time, because roasted peppers have a tendency to bleed their juices when left to rest for an extended period. In either case, be sure to cover the eggs to prevent them from drying out.

Truly Deviled Eggs

Makes 12 pieces

6 eggs
¼ cup Chipotle Mayonnaise (page 58)
1 teaspoon freshly squeezed lime juice
½ teaspoon sea salt
12 cilantro sprigs
¼ to ½ teaspoon cayenne (optional)
1 habanero chile, seeded and finely chopped (optional)

*B*ring 1 quart of water to a boil. Gently lower the eggs into the water with a slotted spoon. Lower the heat and boil the eggs gently for 10 minutes. Remove the eggs with a slotted spoon and immediately plunge them into ice water. Peel the eggs carefully in order to keep them whole. Cut them in half lengthwise and scoop out the yolks.

Chop the yolks thoroughly, and then mash them well with a fork. Stir in the mayonnaise, lime juice, and salt. If the mixture is very dry, stir in a little more mayonnaise.

Scrape the mixture into a pastry bag fitted with a medium to large star tip. Place a cilantro sprig on each egg white half, with the stem sticking down into the cavity and the leaves facing the narrow end. Pipe the yolk mixture into the cavities, dividing it as equally as possible. Sprinkle with the optional cayenne and habanero and serve.

I don't know who came up with the term "deviled" for stuffed eggs, or why, but if the idea has anything to do with that mythical guy whose job it is to cause suffering by fire, then I say let's give the devil his due. Fear not, for the endorphin angel hovereth nearby. If these aren't hot enough for you, dust the tops with cayenne. If they still aren't hot enough for you, chop up an habanero chile and stir it into the yolk mixture and make that endorphin angel earn his wings.

If you haven't made any Chipotle Mayonnaise, take the time now. It's a terrific staple to have in your refrigerator. If you just don't have time or the right ingredients on hand, substitute with plain Udo's Choice Mayonnaise (page 56) and add the optional cayenne and habanero chile. That's if you like spicy food, of course. If you don't, then this recipe is definitely not for you.

Oven-Dried Tomatoes
with Pesto and Brie

Makes 48 pieces

See photo facing page 64

24 or more very small, ripe Roma tomatoes (no longer
than 1½ inches)

½ cup extra-virgin olive oil, more or less as needed

2 tablespoons chopped fresh parsley

4 cloves garlic, pressed or peeled and minced

1 teaspoon sea salt

½ to ¾ teaspoon freshly ground black pepper

½ cup Pesto (page 35), in a paper cornet (see note, page 91)

48 crackers or crostini

½ pound ripe Brie

Preheat the oven to the lowest setting possible, about 185 degrees F.

Line a baking sheet with parchment paper. Cut the tomatoes in half lengthwise and spread them out on the parchment, cut side up. Combine the olive oil, 1½ tablespoons of the parsley, and the garlic in a small bowl, and brush the cut sides of the tomatoes generously with this mixture. Sprinkle the tomatoes with the salt and pepper. Place the tray in the oven and let the tomatoes dry for 8 to 12 hours. Remove from the oven and let cool.

Pipe a layer of the pesto onto each of the crackers or crostini. Lay a thin slice of the Brie, roughly the size of the cracker, over the pesto. Place an oven-dried tomato, cut side up, on the Brie slice. Sprinkle with the remaining parsley and serve.

You know sun-dried tomatoes, right? Same idea. This method is slightly different (no sun required) and a lot faster, but the result is largely the same. With this recipe, the process is stopped before the tomatoes are fully dried, which yields slightly juicy, sweet, strongly flavored dried tomatoes. They won't be shelf stable the way fully dried tomatoes are, but when you start eating them, this won't be an issue, believe me. The rest is pure indulgence, with essential fatty acids thrown in for good measure (and good health!).

If you can't find very small Roma tomatoes, use oversized cherry tomatoes. These are not as fleshy as Romas, but they will dry very nicely in the oven and will have plenty of flavor.

Pesto-Stuffed Cherry Tomatoes

Makes 24 pieces

12 large cherry tomatoes
½ cup Pesto (page 35)
24 very small fresh basil leaves

*C*ut the cherry tomatoes in half crosswise and carefully scoop out and discard the seeds. Turn the halves over onto a paper towel to drain for about 20 minutes. Place the pesto in a pastry bag fitted with a medium star or round tip. Pipe about 1 teaspoon of the pesto into the cavity of each tomato half. Garnish each with a basil leaf and serve immediately, before the basil leaf wilts.

If you want to make these in advance, keep them refrigerated and add the basil leaf garnish just before serving.

If you have any Pesto on hand, these are a snap to prepare. If not, they'll still be very easy and quite delicious.

Hummus-Stuffed Cherry Tomatoes

Makes 24 pieces

12 large cherry tomatoes
1 cup Hummus (page 63)
1 tablespoon chopped fresh parsley

Cut the cherry tomatoes in half crosswise and carefully scoop out and discard the seeds. Turn the halves over onto a paper towel to drain for about 20 minutes. Using a pastry bag fitted with a plain round tip, or a small spoon, fill the tomato halves with the Hummus. Garnish the top of each with some of the parsley and serve.

These are very quick to prepare, especially if you have some fresh Hummus in the refrigerator. They are also quite eye appealing and full of flavor. As a variation, try using Baba Ghanoush (page 62) in place of the Hummus, garnished with a thin slice of kalamata olive and a leaf of parsley. Place the stuffed tomatoes on a banana leaf or nestle them among citrus leaves on a platter, for added effect.

Zucchini Boats
with Roasted Garlic Purée

See photo facing page 64

Makes about 12 pieces

2 or 3 small zucchini

1 red bell pepper, roasted (see note, page 26) and thinly sliced

1 teaspoon Udo's Oil

1 teaspoon finely chopped fresh oregano

$\frac{1}{4}$ teaspoon sea salt

$\frac{1}{4}$ teaspoon freshly ground black pepper

$\frac{1}{3}$ cup Roasted Garlic Purée (page 37)

1 tablespoon chopped fresh parsley

*C*ut the zucchini in half lengthwise. Trim off the ends, then cut them crosswise into equal pieces about $1\frac{1}{2}$ inches long. There should be about 12 pieces in all. Carefully carve out the middle portion of the flesh on each piece to form little boats. Blanch the boats in boiling salted water for 30 to 60 seconds, just until the zucchini are very slightly tender but still crisp enough to hold their shape. Drain and plunge them into ice water to stop the cooking completely. Drain again. Turn them over onto a towel to drain thoroughly for about 20 minutes.

Toss the pepper slices with the Udo's Oil, oregano, salt, and pepper and mix well. Scoop a generous teaspoon of Roasted Garlic Purée into the cavity of each zucchini boat and place it on a tray or platter. Carefully mound some of the roasted pepper mixture on top of the filled boats. Sprinkle with the parsley and serve.

A good zucchini is hard to find. No, that wasn't a naughty remark. All too often farmers allow zucchini to grow to the point where they are huge, and their skin is tough and the flesh is tasteless. For this recipe you'll need to pick the smallest zucchini you can find, preferably no more than an inch in diameter. The rest is easy.

SOUPS

There are few things more satisfying or instantly nourishing than a good soup. It's the ultimate one-dish meal, suitable for any time of day. Fortunately, it's also an excellent vehicle for Udo's Oil, enabling one to get a healthy serving of it with every bowl. In the recipes that follow, you'll find uses for a number of infused oils paired with the soups. In some cases, the oil is added in the form of a sauce, such as Pesto (page 35) or Roasted Red Pepper Sauce (page 30).

The main thing to remember is that since Udo's Oil must never be heated, you should only add it to the portion of soup you're going to eat right away. If you plan to keep leftovers, reserve that portion without the added oil. Then proceed as instructed when reheating the soup at a later time.

Chilled Spicy Avocado Soup

Makes about 8 cups

- 2 tablespoons extra-virgin olive oil
- 2 white onions, minced
- 3 stalks celery, strings removed and minced
- 3 cloves garlic, peeled and minced
- 1 piece (1 inch) fresh ginger, peeled and minced
- 2 jalapeño chiles, seeded and minced
- 1 teaspoon ground coriander
- ¾ teaspoon sea salt
- 1 quart vegetable broth
- 4 fresh tarragon sprigs
- 3 ripe avocados
- 1 tablespoon freshly squeezed lime juice
- ¼ cup Udo's Oil
- 1 tablespoon finely chopped fresh parsley

Serve this in hot weather. Unlike other chilled soups, it will add a pleasant heat as it cools you down. The tarragon flavor will come through miraculously as an ethereal presence.

For extra eye appeal and flavor, drizzle a little Herb Oil (page 25) on the surface of the soup just before sprinkling with the chopped parsley. If you haven't made any Herb Oil, don't let that stop you. Just use plain Udo's Oil and enjoy the soup.

*H*eat the olive oil very gently over low heat in a large, heavy soup pot and add the onions, celery, garlic, ginger, chiles, coriander, and salt and stir well. Cover and let the vegetables sweat for about 10 minutes, stirring often. Add tablespoons of water, as needed, to keep the mixture moist.

Add the broth and the tarragon sprigs. Simmer for 8 to 10 minutes, remove from the heat, and let cool. Remove the tarragon sprigs.

While the soup is cooking, cut the avocados into chunks and toss them with the lime juice. Transfer the avocados to a blender, add the cooled soup, and process until smooth. Strain through a fine mesh sieve and whisk in the Udo's Oil. Cover and refrigerate until cold, at least 3 hours.

Just before serving, whisk thoroughly. Ladle into chilled bowls and garnish with a sprinkling of the parsley.

Curried Carrot Soup with Ginger

Makes about 14 cups

2 tablespoons extra-virgin olive oil

1 large onion, finely diced

10 cloves garlic, peeled and minced

2 tablespoons peeled and very finely minced fresh ginger

8 cups grated carrots

2 tablespoons curry powder

1 teaspoon sea salt

½ teaspoon freshly ground black pepper

8 cups vegetable broth

1 russet potato, peeled and grated

½ cup coarsely chopped fresh cilantro

¼ cup Udo's Oil

½ to 1 cup Scallion Oil (page 28; optional)

*H*eat the olive oil in a heavy pot over moderate heat. Add the onion, garlic, and ginger, stir, and reduce the heat to low. Cover the pot and allow the vegetables to sweat for about 10 minutes, or until very soft and aromatic. Stir in the carrots, curry powder, salt, and pepper. Add the broth and bring to a boil. Add the potato, cover the pot, adjust the heat to maintain a steady low simmer, and cook until the vegetables are very tender, about 45 minutes.

Working in small batches, purée the soup in a blender and strain it back into the pot. If the soup is too thick, add a little more broth or water. Just before serving, turn off the heat and stir in the cilantro and Udo's Oil. Ladle into soup bowls and garnish with a drizzle of Scallion Oil, if desired.

Absolutely delicious. The complex layering of flavors in this soup belies the simplicity of its preparation. Oddly, in spite of its unusual taste, even most children like it.

For a more elegant presentation, use a parchment cornet (see note, page 96) to pipe two thin, concentric circles of Scallion Oil on the surface of the soup, and then draw a toothpick back and forth through them to form a decorative flourish.

Black Bean Soup

Makes about 10 cups

1 pound dried black beans

2 large white onions, finely diced

¼ cup extra-virgin olive oil

¼ cup pasilla chili powder (see note)

2 tablespoons minced garlic

1 teaspoon dried marjoram

4 Roma tomatoes

1 or 2 chipotle chiles en adobo

1 tablespoon sea salt

4 cloves garlic, peeled

2 cups vegetable broth

2 tablespoons freshly squeezed lime juice

½ cup coarsely chopped fresh cilantro

10 tablespoons Simple Garlic Oil (page 22),
    or more as needed

Grated or crumbled Cotija cheese (see note, page 93; optional)

Sort through the beans, discarding any stones or other debris. Wash thoroughly in cold water, drain, cover with fresh water, and soak for 8 to 12 hours. Drain the beans, rinse, and place in a large pot. Add half the onions along with the olive oil, chili powder, minced garlic, marjoram, and enough water to cover by about 2½ inches. Bring to a boil over high heat. Lower the heat to maintain a steady simmer, cover, and cook for 1½ to 2 hours, or until the beans are tender. If you need to add more water, be sure that it is boiling water.

Combine the tomatoes, remaining onions, chiles, salt, and garlic cloves in a blender and process until very smooth.

There are many versions of black bean soup, including this one, which is distinctly Mexican in flavor. In Cuba, the chiles would be absent, replaced by a bay leaf and a splash of dry sherry. If you don't enjoy spicy food, that might be a better option for you. If you elect to try the Cuban version, discard the bay leaf before serving. Stir in the Udo's Oil, but omit the cilantro and Cotija cheese. Serve the soup as is, or add a swirl of heavy cream.

Pasilla is a particular Mexican dried chile with a unique taste that goes especially well with black beans. Look for it in the Hispanic or Mexican section of the store.

Strain through a fine mesh sieve to remove any bits of seeds or skins. Slowly stir into the beans in as thin a stream as possible so the beans don't stop simmering. Continue cooking until the mixture is thick and saucy (this could take from 10 to 45 minutes).

Scoop out about half of the beans and purée them with the broth in batches in a blender. Pour the blended beans back into the pot with the remaining beans and reheat. If the soup is too thick, add a little more broth or water. Remove from the heat and stir in the lime juice. Taste and adjust the seasonings, if needed. Reserve 1 tablespoon of the cilantro and add the remainder to the soup.

To serve, ladle into bowls, stir 1 tablespoon or more of the Simple Garlic Oil into each bowl, and garnish with the reserved cilantro and sprinklings of the Cotija cheese, if using.

Cotija is a sheep's milk cheese, reminiscent of the Greek feta, but drier and much more pungent. In Mexico, it's usually served with beans, tacos, tostadas, and some soups. A fairly good Cotija is now made in California and sold in most American supermarkets. If you can't find this cheese, don't worry about it—the soup itself stands very well on its own.

Mexyssoise

Makes about 16 cups

4 large ears white corn, shucked and silk removed

12 cups water

6 vegetable bouillon cubes

2 pounds tomatillos, dry skins removed and well washed

2 packages (10 ounces each) frozen lima beans

1½ pounds russet potatoes, peeled and coarsely chopped

2 large bunches cilantro, stems included, well washed

1 large bunch parsley, stems included, well washed

1 large white onion, coarsely chopped

10 cloves garlic, peeled

2 poblano chiles, roasted (see note, page 26)

2 or more green serrano chiles

1 teaspoon sea salt

½ teaspoon freshly ground black pepper

½ cup Udo's Oil

1 cup sour cream (optional)

Herb Oil (page 25; optional)

Cut the kernels from the corn and blanch them in boiling salted water until tender-crisp. Drain, refresh in cold water, drain well again, and set aside. Scrape the starch from the corn cobs into a large, heavy soup pot. Add the water and bouillon cubes and bring to a boil. Add the tomatillos, lima beans, and potatoes and bring to a boil. Cover the pot, adjust the heat to maintain a steady low simmer, and cook until the vegetables are very tender, about 30 minutes.

Working in small batches, purée the hot soup in a blender along with the cilantro, parsley, onion, garlic, poblano chiles, serrano chiles, salt, pepper, and Udo's Oil. Strain, return to the pot, and add the reserved corn. If the soup is too thick, add a little more water. Refrigerate until cold. Ladle into soup bowls and garnish with a dollop of sour cream, if using, and a drizzle of Herb Oil, if desired.

This complex and velvety-smooth invention of mine was inspired by the French classic vichyssoise, which is served cold. I had my first taste of vichyssoise under an umbrella by a hotel pool in, of all places, Peru. Whereas gazpacho had always struck me as more like tomato juice with chopped up salad in it, this was a genuine soup, but cold! On a hot day it seemed perfect. The raw ingredients in this version accentuate the qualities of a cold soup. However, this same soup has also been well received when served hot. The addition of cooked white corn kernels at the end provides further textural interest.

For a more elegant presentation, use a parchment cornet (see note, page 96) to pipe two thin, concentric circles of the Herb Oil on the surface of the soup, and then draw a toothpick back and forth through them to form a decorative flourish. If using the sour cream, pipe two additional circles, alternating between the oil circles before drawing the toothpick through, for an even more stunning effect.

Minestrone

Makes about 20 cups

2 tablespoons extra-virgin olive oil

1 large onion, diced

12 cloves garlic, peeled and sliced

8 cups vegetable broth

2 cups peeled, seeded, and chopped tomatoes

2 cups peeled and diced pumpkin or butternut squash

2 cups coarsely chopped red Swiss chard

2 cups cut green beans, cut in $1/2$-inch pieces

8 stalks celery, strings removed and diced

4 carrots, diced

4 zucchini, diced

2 large potatoes, diced

1 cup diced broccoli stems

1 cup shelled green peas

$1/2$ cup coarsely chopped fresh parsley

1 teaspoon sea salt

$1/2$ teaspoon freshly ground black pepper

2 cups cooked cannellini beans or white navy beans

2 to 6 tablespoons Pesto (page 35)

*H*eat the olive oil in a heavy pot over moderate heat. Add the onion and garlic, stir, and reduce the heat to low. Cover the pot and allow the vegetables to sweat for about 10 minutes, or until very soft and aromatic. Add the broth, tomatoes, pumpkin, Swiss chard, green beans, celery, carrots, zucchini, potatoes, broccoli stems, peas, parsley, salt, and pepper. Bring to a boil, then immediately adjust the heat to maintain a steady low simmer. Cook until the vegetables are very tender, about $1\frac{1}{2}$ hours. Add the cannellini beans and cook 15 minutes longer.

Just before serving, remove the pot from the heat and stir in the Pesto to taste.

The addition of Pesto at the end will take your minestrone to a different dimension. No one will be able to put their finger on it, but the soup will have a unique, underlying presence of basil and cheese. This is a crowd pleaser. Young and old will swoon, guaranteed.

Corn Soup with Roasted Peppers

Makes about 10 cups

See photo facing page 97

2 tablespoons extra-virgin olive oil

1 large onion, finely diced

10 cloves garlic, peeled and minced

1 teaspoon sea salt

½ teaspoon freshly ground black pepper

8 cups vegetable broth

8 cups fresh or frozen corn kernels

1 red bell pepper, roasted (see note, page 26) and diced

1 green bell pepper, roasted (see note, page 26) and diced

¼ cup Udo's Oil

4 scallions, finely sliced

Heat the olive oil in a heavy pot over moderate heat. Add the onion, garlic, salt, and pepper, stir, and reduce the heat to low. Cover the pot and allow the vegetables to sweat for about 10 minutes, or until very soft and aromatic. Add the broth and bring to a boil. Add the corn and lower the heat. Cover the pot, adjust the heat to maintain a steady low simmer, and cook until the corn is very tender, about 30 minutes. Scoop out about 1½ cups of the corn with a slotted spoon and set aside.

Working in small batches, purée the soup in a blender, strain, and discard the tough skins. Return to the pot and add the reserved corn and roasted peppers. If the soup is too thick, add a little more broth. Just before serving, turn off the heat and stir in the Udo's Oil and scallions. Ladle into soup bowls and serve at once.

Photo: Bitter Melon Salad (page 115)

Most people will swear there is cream in this soup, although there isn't even any milk. Even hard-core meat eaters will enjoy this. Kids love it.

For a more elegant presentation, fill a parchment cornet (see box below) with Scallion Oil (page 28) and pipe two thin, concentric circles on the surface of the soup, then draw a toothpick back and forth through them to form a decorative flourish.

Parchment Cornets

To make a parchment cornet, cut a large triangular piece of parchment paper (baking parchment), join the corners to form a cone with a tightly closed tip, and crimp the corners together to secure them in place. Prop up the cones by placing them in a tall glass and fill them about two-thirds full. Fold the top to enclose the filling and cut a small opening in the tip. Gently squeeze from the top to pipe the filling in a thin stream for use as a decorative garnish.

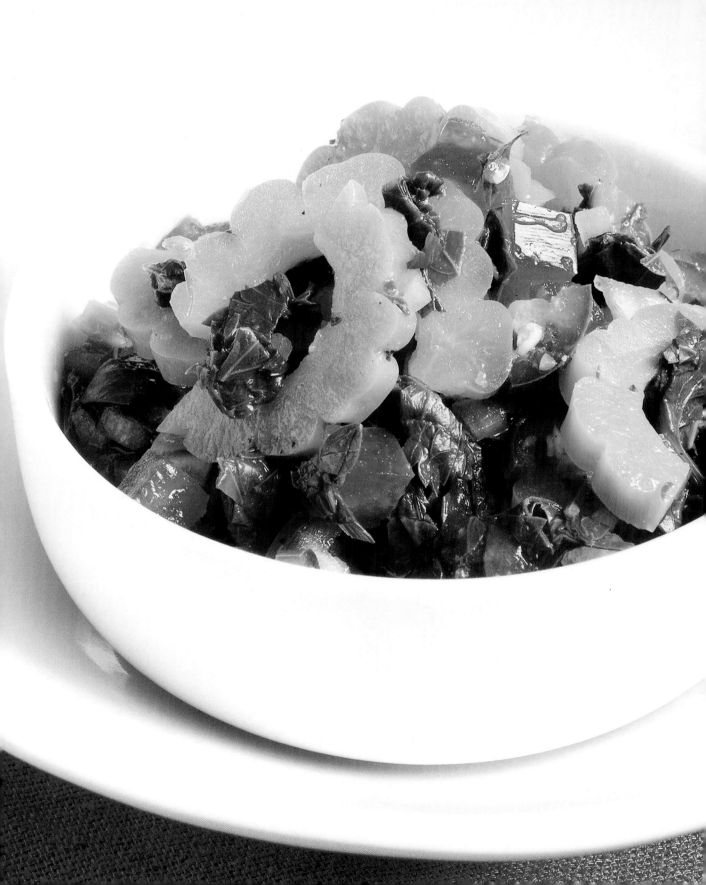

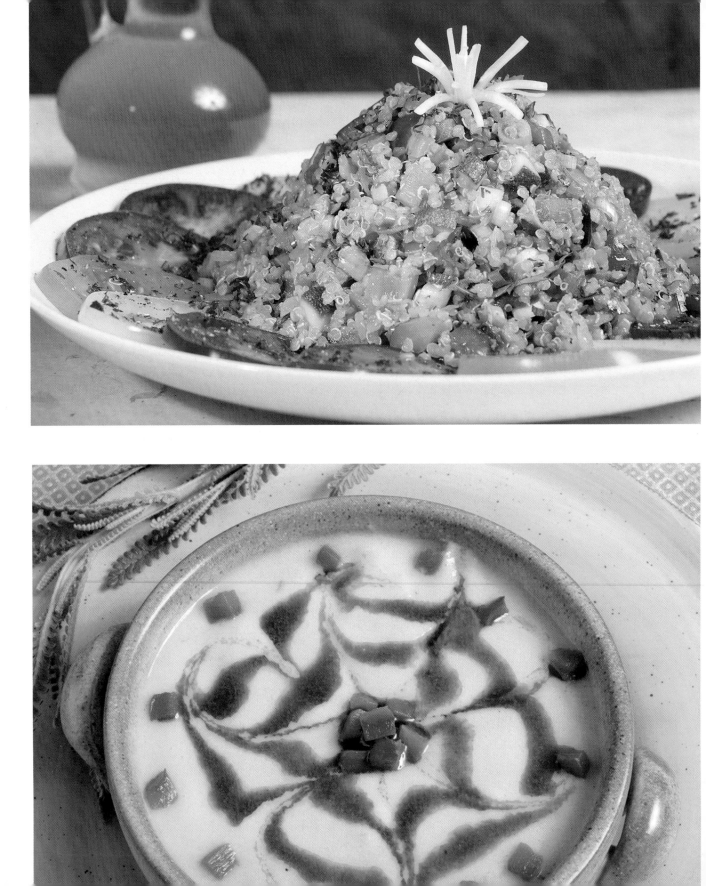

Creamy Garlic Soup

Makes about 10 cups

- 4 heads elephant garlic, peeled and root ends cut off
- 1 quart vegetable broth
- 2 leeks, white part only, thinly sliced
- 1 large russet potato, peeled and diced
- 1 teaspoon sea salt
- 1½ teaspoons freshly ground black pepper
- Pinch of ground mace, plus more for garnish
- ¼ cup Udo's Oil
- Scallion Oil (page 28; optional)
- 1 tablespoon snipped chives

*B*lanch the garlic cloves in boiling water for 1 minute, drain, and refresh under cold water. Repeat this process 3 more times. Chop the garlic coarsely and put it in a heavy saucepan along with the broth, leeks, potato, and ½ teaspoon of the salt. Bring to a boil, then lower the heat to maintain a steady simmer. Cover and cook for 30 minutes or longer, until the vegetables are very tender.

Working in small batches, purée the soup in a blender and strain it back into the pot. It should have a creamy texture, but if the soup is too thick, add just a little more broth. Add the remaining salt along with the pepper and mace to taste and reheat.

Remove from the heat and whisk in the Udo's Oil. Ladle into soup bowls. If desired, place a large drop of Scallion Oil in the center of each bowl and pull a toothpick out from the center in several places to form a starburst. Garnish with a sprinkling of the snipped chives and a very light dusting of mace.

Photo: Quinoa Pilaf (page 149),
Corn Soup with Roasted Peppers (page 96)

Don't skip the blanching steps, whatever you do, or your friends will never forgive you. The flavor and intensity of the garlic will mellow by repeated blanching and refreshing. In France, a mild but fragrant garlic purée is made by blanching the garlic in milk, which you may wish to try for this soup. If you're making the Scallion Oil for this occasion, don't strain it; whisk it briefly before serving to suspend the solids, which will give it a creamy texture and provide a pleasant contrast to the white soup.

Creamy Gingered Cabbage Soup

Makes about 12 cups

2 tablespoons extra-virgin olive oil

2 large onions, diced

1 green cabbage, diced

½ red cabbage, diced

¼ cup peeled and thinly sliced garlic

1 to 2 teaspoons sea salt

2 quarts vegetable broth

2 tablespoons peeled and grated fresh ginger

¼ cup Udo's Oil

Herb Oil (page 25; optional)

¼ cup snipped chives

The illusion of cream comes from the mere blending of cooked vegetables with Udo's Oil. A jab of ginger perks this soup up enough so that even people who aren't terribly keen on cabbage will enjoy it.

*H*eat the olive oil in a heavy pot over moderate heat. Add the onions, green cabbage, and red cabbage. Stir and reduce the heat to low. Cover the pot and allow the vegetables to sweat for about 10 minutes, or until very soft and aromatic. Stir in the garlic and 1 teaspoon of the salt. Add the broth and bring to a boil. Cover the pot, adjust the heat to maintain a steady low simmer, and cook until the vegetables are very tender, about 45 minutes. Squeeze as much of the juice out of the grated ginger as possible. Discard the solids and add the juice to the soup during the last 10 minutes of cooking.

Scoop out half of the vegetables with a slotted spoon and set aside. Working in small batches, purée the remaining soup in a blender and strain it back into the pot. It should have a creamy texture, but if the soup is too thick, add a little more broth. Scoop out about 1 cup of the blended soup, place it in a small bowl, whisk in the Udo's Oil, and cover to keep warm. Stir the reserved vegetables into the pot and reheat. Taste and add more salt, if needed. Just before serving, turn off the heat and stir in the soup and oil mixture. Ladle into soup bowls and garnish with a drizzle of the Herb Oil, if desired, and a sprinkling of the snipped chives.

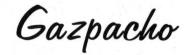

Gazpacho

Makes about 16 cups

1 quart tomato-based vegetable juice blend or plain tomato juice

3 cups tomato purée (preferably Italian *passata di pomodoro*)

2 green bell peppers, roasted (see note, page 26)
    and finely diced

2 red bell peppers, roasted (see note, page 26) and finely diced

2 yellow bell peppers, roasted (see note, page 26)
    and finely diced

2 stalks celery, strings removed and minced

2 bunches scallions, very thinly sliced

2 tablespoons coarsely chopped fresh tarragon

2 tablespoons finely chopped fresh parsley

2 to 4 cloves garlic, peeled and minced

1/2 cup Udo's Oil

1/4 cup freshly squeezed lemon juice

1 teaspoon sea salt

1/2 teaspoon freshly ground black pepper

*P*ut the vegetable juice blend and tomato purée in a large bowl and stir in the roasted peppers, celery, scallions, tarragon, parsley, and garlic. In a small bowl, whisk together the oil, lemon juice, salt, and pepper and stir this mixture into the soup. Let it rest for several minutes, then taste and adjust the seasonings, adding more salt, pepper, or lemon juice, if desired. Chill thoroughly before serving.

A fabulous summer dish, gazpacho is refreshing and nourishing; it's also an excellent appetizer. I served this to a charming, attractive woman once. Not counting the margaritas, it was the first dish of mine she had ever tasted. We're married now.

Fava Bean Soup

Makes about 10 cups

- 2 tablespoons extra-virgin olive oil
- 2 medium white onions, finely diced
- 2 stalks celery, strings removed and finely diced
- 7 cloves garlic, peeled and minced
- 6 cups vegetable broth
- 1 or 2 green serrano chiles, finely chopped
- 2 pounds shelled fava beans
- 1 teaspoon sea salt
- ½ teaspoon freshly ground black pepper
- 2 bunches fresh cilantro, washed and wrung dry in a towel (about 3 cups, packed)
- ⅓ cup Udo's Oil
- 1 tablespoon finely chopped fresh parsley

*H*eat the olive oil in a heavy pot over moderate heat. Add the onions, celery, and garlic, stir, and reduce the heat to low. Cover the pot and allow the vegetables to sweat for about 10 minutes, or until very soft and aromatic. Add the broth and chiles and bring to a boil. Remove several small fava beans and set them aside to use as a garnish, then add the fava beans, salt, and pepper and stir well. When the soup returns to a boil, adjust the heat to maintain a steady low simmer, and cook for 25 minutes or longer, until the vegetables and beans are very tender.

Working in small batches, purée the soup in a blender along with the cilantro and strain it back into the pot. If the soup is too thick, add a little more broth. Reheat the soup. Taste and adjust the seasonings, if needed. Just before serving, turn off the heat and stir in the Udo's Oil. Ladle into soup bowls and garnish with the reserved small fava beans and a light sprinkling of the parsley.

Fava beans are an Italian-Mediterranean passion for sure, but in Mexico they're quite popular as well, notably in the form of this soup. Unfortunately, they turn a sad olive color when cooked long enough to purée, but I bring back that bright green color by blending them with cilantro at the end. Just in the nick of time, so to speak. Now that fava beans have come into their own in the United States and Canada, they can be found frozen in many supermarkets as well as in the produce section. This is one instance where frozen produce will give identical results as fresh, so save yourself a ton of work and buy the frozen ones.

Potato-Leek Soup with Rosemary

Makes about 12 cups

8 cups vegetable broth

3 leeks, cut into ½-inch dice

4 small to medium russet potatoes, peeled, quartered, and very thinly sliced

2 cloves garlic, peeled and minced

1 teaspoon sea salt

½ teaspoon freshly ground black or white pepper

¼ cup Rosemary Oil (page 27)

¼ cup snipped chives

*P*lace the broth, leeks, potatoes, garlic, salt, and pepper in a heavy soup pot. Bring to a boil over high heat, stir, and adjust the heat to maintain a steady low simmer. Cover and cook for 35 to 40 minutes, or until very tender. Scoop out about one-third of the vegetables and set aside.

Working in small batches, purée the soup in a blender and strain it back into the pot. If the soup is too thick, add a little more broth. Add the reserved vegetables and reheat. Just before serving, turn off the heat and stir in the Rosemary Oil. Ladle into soup bowls and garnish with the chives.

This is a good soup for winter months, not only because leeks remain plentiful, but because of its warming qualities. It's strictly comfort food, yet suitable for even discriminating gourmets. The rosemary aromatic is a natural partner with potatoes.

Pumpkin Soup

Makes about 16 cups

2 tablespoons extra-virgin olive oil

1 large onion, finely diced

12 cloves garlic, peeled and minced

8 cups vegetable broth

1 small pumpkin (about 4 pounds) peeled, seeded, and cut in 1/2-inch pieces

1 teaspoon sea salt

1/2 teaspoon freshly ground black pepper

1/2 teaspoon ground allspice

1 cup freshly grated Parmesan cheese

1/4 cup Udo's Oil

Curry Oil (page 24; optional)

*H*eat the olive oil in a heavy pot over moderate heat. Add the onion and garlic, stir, and reduce the heat to low. Cover the pot and allow the vegetables to sweat for about 10 minutes, or until very soft and aromatic. Add the broth and bring to a boil. Add the pumpkin, salt, pepper, and allspice, cover, and adjust the heat to maintain a steady low simmer. Cook until the vegetables are very tender, about 45 minutes.

Working in small batches, purée the soup in a blender with the Parmesan cheese. Strain, return the soup to the pot, and reheat. If the soup is too thick, add a little more broth. Just before serving, turn off the heat and whisk in the Udo's Oil. Ladle into soup bowls and garnish with a drizzle of Curry Oil, if desired.

If you entertain guests who think they don't like squash or pumpkin, don't tell them what's in the soup; just let them start eating. Wait until they ask what it is, then blow their minds with the news. It's one of those moments cooks live for. If you're serving people who do like pumpkin, they'll probably guess, but so what?

As a simple variation, replace the pumpkin with an equal quantity of butternut squash. For a vegan dish, simply omit the Parmesan cheese.

For a more elegant presentation, use a parchment cornet (see note, page 96) to pipe two thin, concentric circles of the Curry Oil on the surface of the soup, and then draw a toothpick back and forth through them to form a decorative flourish.

Roasted Red and Yellow Pepper Soup

Makes about 12 cups

¼ cup extra-virgin olive oil

2 cups chopped onions

1 cup diced carrots

½ cup diced celery

7 cloves garlic, peeled and chopped

8 cups vegetable broth

2 russet potatoes, peeled and diced

1 rosemary sprig

1 bay leaf

1 teaspoon sea salt

½ teaspoon freshly ground black pepper

4 yellow bell peppers, roasted (see note, page 26)

4 red bell peppers, roasted (see note, page 26)

Dash of Tabasco sauce

½ cup Udo's Oil

¼ to ⅓ cup Herb Oil (page 25)

The contrasting colors of the two peppers make a dramatic presentation, but the flavors are rather different too, so encourage your guests to use their spoons judiciously in order to scoop up both types of peppers and experience the soup to its maximum taste potential. Roasting the peppers on the spot is preferable, but you can obtain quite acceptable results using roasted peppers from a jar. Just be sure to rinse them well before proceeding with the recipe.

*W*arm the olive oil in a large pan and stir in the onions, carrots, celery, garlic, and 1 tablespoon of the broth. Adjust the heat to the lowest setting, cover, and let the vegetables sweat for about 10 minutes, stirring often and adding small amounts of broth, if needed, to keep the mixture moist. Add the remaining broth, potatoes, rosemary sprig, bay leaf, salt, and pepper. Simmer for about 30 minutes, or until the vegetables are very soft.

Remove the rosemary sprig and bay leaf and purée the soup in batches in a blender. Strain. Blend half of the soup with the red bell peppers and season with Tabasco sauce to taste. Blend the other half of the soup with the yellow bell peppers. Keep the two soups separate. Taste and adjust the seasonings, if needed.

To serve, heat the two soups separately. Remove from the heat and whisk ¼ cup of the Udo's Oil into each soup. Carefully pour the two soups into individual soup bowls simultaneously, from opposite sides, so that the colors remain separate as much as possible. Use the back of a spoon to swirl one into the other to achieve a yin-yang effect. Using a parchment cornet (see note, page 96), pipe a line of Herb Oil along the juncture of the two soups. Add contrasting dots of the opposing soups to complete the look. If this seems a little hokey to you, just pour the soups to keep the two colors separate and garnish with Herb Oil.

Red Bean Soup

1 pound dried red beans

4 tablespoons extra-virgin olive oil

2 bay leaves

4 large tomatoes, coarsely chopped

2 large onions, finely diced

21 cloves garlic, peeled

2 teaspoons sea salt

2 carrots, finely diced

2 stalks celery, strings removed and finely diced

1 potato, finely diced

1 red bell pepper, roasted (see note, page 26) and finely diced

7 cloves garlic, peeled and thinly sliced

2 cups vegetable broth

1 bunch cilantro, coarsely chopped

1/3 cup Udo's Oil

2 tablespoons freshly squeezed lime juice

1/3 to 1/2 cup Basil Oil (page 22)

Sort through the red beans, discarding any stones or other debris. Wash thoroughly in cold water and drain. Cover with fresh water by about 3 inches and soak for 8 to 12 hours.

Drain the beans, rinse, and place in a large pot. Add 3 tablespoons of the olive oil, the bay leaves, and enough water to cover by about 2½ inches. Bring to a boil over high heat. Cover and reduce the heat to maintain a steady simmer. Cook for 1½ to 2 hours, or until tender. If you need to add more water, be sure to add boiling water.

This is much more than a red version of Black Bean Soup (page 92), as you'll see. The diced vegetables give it a world of surprising taste and a lot of texture variety, secreted in the cloak of a rich red bean purée. It's just a wonderful thing to eat. At Indian grocery stores, look for *rajma dal,* which is the Indian red bean. It's slightly smaller, a deeper red, and much tastier than American red beans.

Combine the tomatoes, half of the onions, the 21 cloves of garlic, and the salt in a blender and process until smooth. Add to the beans slowly, in as thin a stream as possible, so the beans don't stop simmering. Cook until the mixture is reduced to a sauce. Discard the bay leaves.

Pour the remaining 1 tablespoon olive oil into a large pot and add the remaining onion and the carrots and celery. Place over very low heat and cook, stirring constantly, for 5 to 10 minutes, until the vegetables are aromatic. Stir in the potato, bell pepper, and sliced garlic. Add the vegetable broth, cover, and cook gently until the vegetables are tender, about 10 minutes. Strain the broth into a bowl, reserving the vegetables. Purée half of the beans with the broth in a blender until smooth. Return to the pot and add the vegetables and remaining beans. Stir well, taste, and adjust the seasonings, if needed. Reserve 2 tablespoons of the cilantro for garnish and add the rest to the soup, stirring well.

To serve, reheat the soup, stirring often to prevent sticking. Remove from the heat and add the Udo's Oil and lime juice, stirring well. Ladle into bowls and garnish with the reserved cilantro and a flourish of the Basil Oil. Serve at once.

Zucchinissoise

Makes about 6 servings

1 tablespoon extra-virgin olive oil

2 white onions, thinly sliced

2 leeks, thinly sliced

6 cups vegetable broth

1 large russet potato, peeled and grated (see note)

1 teaspoon sea salt

½ teaspoon freshly ground black pepper

4 small to medium zucchini, grated

⅓ cup Basil Oil (page 22)

2 tablespoons snipped chives

Heat the olive oil in a heavy pot over moderate heat. Add the onions and leeks, stir, and reduce the heat to low. Cover the pot and allow the vegetables to sweat for about 10 minutes, or until very soft and aromatic. Add the broth, potato, salt, and pepper and bring to a boil. Cover the pot, adjust the heat to maintain a steady low simmer, and cook until tender, about 30 minutes. Add the zucchini and cook 10 minutes longer, or until the zucchini is very soft.

Working in small batches, purée the soup in a blender and strain it back into the pot. It should have a creamy texture, but if the soup is too thick, add a little more broth. Taste and adjust the seasonings, if needed, and reheat. Ladle into soup bowls and garnish with a light drizzle of the Basil Oil and a sprinkling of the snipped chives.

Here's another twist on the old French classic— I came up with this one when I was trying to use some zucchini I had carved up to make garnishes for something else. The poor things were so defaced, a purée was all they were good for. As it turned out, the soup was every bit as good as the original dish that had caused me to savage the zucchini. So I had actually created the mother of my own invention. I love this job!

If you don't have any Basil Oil prepared, add about 8 fresh basil leaves to the soup during the blending process. Then, just before serving, remove the soup from the heat and whisk in ¼ cup plain Udo's Oil. Garnish with the chives and serve.

To prevent discoloration, peel and grate the potato just before using.

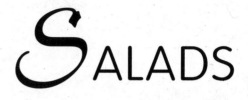

SALADS

No doubt about it, the way to get the most out of our food is to eat it raw. I know this is an odd thing for someone who has made a good living from cooking to be saying, but all evidence supports it. In some of the salads that follow, a few of the ingredients will be subjected to some minor cooking in order to improve their taste, texture, or ability to combine readily with other ingredients. The net result, however, is that more raw food will ultimately appear in your diet, having been made more agreeable to the palate.

The many salad dressings in this book also help keep raw food from becoming a bore. In some cases, such as Udo's Caesar Salad (page 132), I have included the salad dressing in the salad recipe, simply because the dressing has virtually no other application. In most, however, I have listed the most suitable dressing in the list of ingredients. Although this may seem inconvenient, it is intentional, because the dressings themselves have many applications and should be presented as important preparations in their own right. Having them in their own section of the book highlights them as valuable resources in our effort to include the right fats in our diet every day.

Apple and Fennel Salad with Saint Agûr

Makes 4 servings

See photo facing page 129

2 large fennel bulbs

2 large Granny Smith apples

2 tablespoons freshly squeezed lemon juice

¼ cup Udo's Oil

¼ teaspoon sea salt

¼ teaspoon freshly ground black pepper

4 cups baby romaine leaves

4 thick slices Saint Agûr cheese or Gorgonzola
    (about 1 to 2 ounces each)

¼ cup lightly crushed pecans

2 tablespoons snipped chives

Cut each fennel bulb in half lengthwise, carve out and discard the tough inner core, and thinly slice the fennel crosswise. Peel and quarter the apples and remove the seeds and stems. Slice the quarters crosswise, a little thinner than ¼ inch. Whisk the lemon juice, oil, salt, and pepper together and toss with the apple and fennel.

Divide the lettuce leaves among four plates. Toss the salad again and place a mound on each bed of lettuce. Rest a slice of the cheese against one side of the salad and sprinkle 1 tablespoon of the pecans over it. Sprinkle the dish with the snipped chives and serve.

The combination of blue cheeses with apples or pears is a time-tested delicious one. Saint Agûr, a French blue cheese similar to the Italian Gorgonzola, is unsurpassed for this particular pairing. It has a unique composition of creamy, sweet, acidic, and pungent qualities that blend beautifully with the fresh taste of a crisp green apple. In this salad, fennel and pecans add additional layers of texture and taste complexity. The dressing is pure simplicity, allowing the main characters to assert themselves fully.

Baby Squash Salad

Makes 4 servings

1 large or 2 small heads Boston lettuce

1 pound assorted baby squashes (whatever varieties are
available)

¼ cup aged balsamic vinegar (see note)

¼ cup Simple Garlic Oil (page 22; see note)

¼ teaspoon sea salt

¼ teaspoon freshly ground black pepper

1 small red onion, finely slivered

1½ cups very small cherry tomatoes

1 tablespoon coarsely chopped fresh basil leaves

*B*reak up the heads of lettuce, leaving the inner leaves
whole. Wash and spin or pat dry. Blanch the squashes in
boiling salted water for 1 minute, drain, refresh under cold
water, and spread out on a towel to dry. Cut each squash in
half lengthwise.

Whisk together the balsamic vinegar, oil, salt, and pepper
in a large bowl. Taste for tartness. If it seems too tart for
your palate, add a little more oil. Add the squashes and
onion and toss.

To serve, make a bed of lettuce on each plate. Toss the
squashes again and divide them among the plates, mound-
ing them in the center of the bed of lettuce. Garnish with the
cherry tomatoes and a little of the basil.

If you haven't made any Simple Garlic Oil, this
is a good time to do it. But if you don't really
like garlic, go ahead and use plain Udo's Oil.
On this salad, the garlic isn't crucial.

All too often squashes are allowed to grow to
monstrous proportions, at a terrible cost to the quality of the
vegetable. At that point, the once-tender squash is virtually
all water and no taste, the skin is thick and tough, and the
seeds are overgrown and gristly. Baby squashes are
quite the reverse, with firm flesh and highly concentrated
flavor. They have a pleasant sweet taste, with a very slight
bitterness in the skin. Aged balsamic vinegar is the ideal
complement to these seemingly opposite tastes,
accenting the sweet and taming the bitter.

Aged balsamic vinegar is left to mature for at least
twelve years and has a near-mystical quality that simply
cannot be duplicated. However, since it is both
difficult to find and extremely expensive, you may opt to
commit the cardinal sin of boiling regular commercial
balsamic vinegar until it is reduced to almost a syrup to
obtain a vaguely similar consistency if not the deep rich
flavor. It's better than nothing, but please don't rat me out to
the Italians.

Beet and Barley Salad

Makes about 6 servings

½ cup hulled barley

2 cups vegetable broth

3 large beets, cut into ½-inch dice

1 large tangelo

⅓ cup freshly squeezed Meyer lemon juice (see note)

1 tablespoon red wine vinegar

4 whole cloves

1 bay leaf

½ teaspoon sea salt

½ teaspoon freshly ground black pepper

5 small red onions, thinly sliced (about 1½ to 2 cups)

4 cloves garlic, peeled and thinly sliced

¼ cup Udo's Oil

3 stalks celery, strings removed and finely diced

1 fennel bulb, cored and finely diced

1 bunch scallions, thinly sliced diagonally

1 carrot, grated

¼ cup chopped Italian parsley

½ cup celery leaves

For people who may have the idea that barley is slimy, boring, and tasteless, this is one effective way to alter that perception. In the pleasant company of a citrus-based dressing and all those crunchy, flavorful vegetables, barley acquires a whole new identity.

Meyer lemons are sweeter and less acidic than most other lemons. If you can't find any, don't worry about it. Just use ordinary lemons and add a bit more oil, if needed, to balance the acidity.

*P*lace the barley and broth in a small pot and bring to a boil. Lower the heat and simmer until tender, about 45 minutes. Steam the beets until tender-crisp. Remove them from the steamer and let cool completely.

Grate the zest from the tangelo, cover (to keep it from drying out), and set aside. Squeeze the juice from the tangelo into a saucepan. Add the lemon juice, vinegar, cloves, bay leaf, salt, and pepper. Bring to a boil, reduce the heat, and simmer for 2 to 3 minutes. Add the onions and garlic.

Bring to a simmer and cook for about 1 minute, until just barely softened. Remove from the heat and let cool. Remove and discard the bay leaf and cloves. Strain the liquid into a small bowl (reserve the onions and garlic) and whisk in the oil to make a light dressing. Taste and adjust the seasonings, if needed.

Combine the reserved onions and garlic with the barley, beets, reserved tangelo zest, celery, fennel, scallions, carrot, and parsley. Whisk the dressing again and toss with the vegetables. Refrigerate until ready to serve. Serve in bowls or on a bed of mixed greens, garnished with the celery leaves.

Mixed Bean Salad

Makes 8 to 12 servings

2 cups diced tomatoes
1½ cups diced red onions
1½ cups diced celery
1½ cups peeled and diced jicama
1½ cups diced green bell peppers
1 cup shelled edamame, blanched until tender-crisp
1 cup cooked black beans
1 cup cooked navy beans
1 cup cooked kidney beans
1 cup cooked adzuki beans
1 cup cooked mung beans
1 cup cooked pinto beans
1 cup coarsely chopped fresh cilantro, packed
1½ to 2 cups Roasted Garlic Vinaigrette (page 48)

*C*ombine all the ingredients in a large bowl and toss well. Serve in small bowls or on plates over a bed of lettuce.

The most important ingredient in this salad, oddly enough, isn't one of the beans—you can substitute any of them—it's the jicama. I had made this same dish without jicama countless times before it occurred to me to throw it in. There's something about the satisfying, juicy crunch amid the tender beans that does wonders for this salad.

Belgian Endive Salad with Raspberries

Makes 4 servings

6 Belgian endives
½ cup Raspberry Vinaigrette (page 47)
1 cup raspberries
1 tablespoon snipped chives
¼ cup fresh chervil leaves, loosely packed

*C*arefully trim the endives, separating the leaves but keeping them whole. Discard any bruised or discolored pieces.

To serve, toss the endive leaves in a large bowl with the vinaigrette. Add half of the raspberries and chives. Toss again, very gently. Divide among 4 plates, garnish with the remaining raspberries and chives and the chervil leaves. Serve at once, before the salad wilts.

The characteristic bitter edge of endive is countered nicely by a fruity dressing in this very easy, beautiful salad. Due to its lightness and bright taste, it makes a terrific appetizer. Make an effort to get fresh green chervil, but don't be concerned if you can't find any; although it definitely adds something special to the overall taste experience, this salad will shine perfectly without it.

Bitter Melon Salad

Makes 4 small servings   *See photo facing page 96*

4 medium bitter melons, or 8 small Indian karela
2 bunches fresh fenugreek
⅓ cup Udo's Oil
¼ cup freshly squeezed lemon juice
½ teaspoon sea salt
¼ teaspoon freshly ground black pepper
1 red onion, finely diced
1 large ripe tomato, cut into ½-inch dice
1 fresh green chile, finely chopped (optional)

Split the bitter melons in half lengthwise and scrape out the seeds with the tip of a spoon. Slice them fairly thinly (about ⅛-inch-thick slices) into little arcs. Bring about 1 quart of water to a boil and blanch the melon slices for about 2 minutes, until tender-crisp. Scoop out with a slotted spoon and let cool. Keep the water boiling. Remove and discard the coarse stems from the fenugreek and blanch the leaves in the same water for about 30 seconds. Drain and immediately plunge into ice water to stop the cooking completely. Drain thoroughly in a colander, squeezing out the excess water. Chop the fenugreek coarsely. (Don't throw out the cooking water—drink it!)

Whisk together the oil, lemon juice, salt, and pepper in a large bowl. Add the bitter melon, fenugreek, onion, tomato, and optional chile and toss well. Serve in small bowls as a first course to your most adventurous friends.

> If you prefer, steam the bitter melon rather than boiling it. This will preserve more of the nutrients. Afterward, use the steaming water to blanch the fenugreek.

Bitter melon is one of those foods you either love or hate. It has a very bitter taste (hence the name), but it does grow on you if you can deal with the initial shock. It is extremely good for you. In Chinese medicine it's referred to as "bitter cucumber" and is used as a medicinal herb for treating all sorts of ailments, including diabetes and anemia. You'll find the best variety at Indian grocery stores, where it's known as *karela*.

While you're there, also ask for *methi*, which is fenugreek (make sure you indicate fresh leaves, not the seeds). It looks a bit like a cross between cilantro and clover. Both bitter melon and fenugreek are powerful blood purifiers and tonics. This particular salad has the added advantage of perking up the appetite. Once you acquire the taste for it, you'll be hooked for life.

Asian Coleslaw

Makes 4 to 6 servings

1 tablespoon Japanese sesame oil (see note)

3 tablespoons Udo's Oil

1/2 cup soy sauce

3 tablespoons freshly squeezed lime juice

2 tablespoons balsamic vinegar

2 tablespoons honey

2 cups sliced Chinese cabbage

1 cup julienned snow peas

2 stalks celery, strings removed, cut in half lengthwise,
    and thinly sliced diagonally

1 fennel bulb, cored and thinly sliced

4 scallions, sliced diagonally

2 Thai red chiles, thinly sliced (optional)

2 tablespoons sesame seeds

Whisk together the sesame oil and Udo's Oil. Add the soy sauce, lime juice, balsamic vinegar, and honey and whisk until well blended. Add the cabbage, snow peas, celery, fennel, scallions, optional chiles, and sesame seeds. Toss thoroughly and serve at once.

Serve this as an appetizer (at which it excels) or as part of a buffet. It's also good as a picnic item—even after it has wilted somewhat, it will retain considerable crunch and all of its bright flavors.

Julienne is the culinary term for a particular method of cutting ingredients that results in long, thin strips. An example of this method is thinly slicing a vegetable diagonally, stacking the slices, and then slicing them lengthwise into uniform sticks. This is done both for eye appeal and to ensure even cooking.

Japanese sesame oil (also known as toasted sesame oil) is made from toasted sesame seeds, which give the oil a dark color and rich, somewhat smoky flavor. Not typically used as a cooking oil, it is added sparingly to finished dishes as a flavoring.

Cucumber and Green Olive Salad

Makes 4 servings

2 hothouse cucumbers

2 to 3 teaspoons sea salt, plus an additional $1/4$ teaspoon

1 green bell pepper

1 cup pitted green olives, coarsely chopped

$1/4$ cup chopped fresh mint

$1/4$ cup chopped fresh cilantro

3 tablespoons Udo's Oil

3 tablespoons extra-virgin olive oil

2 tablespoons freshly squeezed lemon juice

1 teaspoon cayenne

$1/4$ teaspoon freshly ground black pepper

*P*eel the cucumbers, cut them in half lengthwise, and scrape out the seeds. Cut into $1/8$-inch-thick slices, sprinkle lightly with 2 to 3 teaspoons of the salt, and allow the slices to drain for about 20 minutes in a colander. Rinse well, then spread out on a towel and pat dry.

Quarter the pepper, remove the seeds and membranes, and cut into thin strips. Place in a bowl with the cucumbers, the remaining $1/4$ teaspoon salt, and all of the remaining ingredients. Toss well, taste, and adjust the seasonings, if needed. Serve at once in small bowls.

This is a spicy salad. If you prefer it less spicy, substitute Hungarian hot paprika for the cayenne. Use only high-quality, large, fleshy green olives for this dish.

Curried Coleslaw

Makes 4 to 6 servings

1 pound red cabbage, thinly sliced or shredded

3 to 4 stalks celery, strings removed, cut in half lengthwise,
    and thinly sliced diagonally

1 carrot, grated

1 fennel bulb, cored and thinly sliced

2 tablespoons fresh ginger, peeled and cut into very fine julienne

2 teaspoons kosher salt

1/2 teaspoon celery seeds

1/4 teaspoon crushed fennel seeds

1/4 cup rice vinegar

1/4 cup Udo's Oil

3 tablespoons honey

1 tablespoon curry powder

1/4 teaspoon freshly ground black pepper

Replacing that sugary mayonnaise with an exotically seasoned vinaigrette results in unexpected flavors. This is a brave new slaw.

Combine the cabbage, celery, carrot, fennel, and ginger in a bowl. Add the salt, celery seeds, and fennel seeds and toss. Let stand for 1 to 4 hours, until wilted. Pour off the liquid.

Whisk together the vinegar, oil, honey, curry powder, and pepper in a large bowl. Add the drained vegetable mixture and toss. Taste and adjust the seasonings, if needed. Cover and refrigerate until ready to serve.

Edamame Salad

Makes 6 to 8 servings

1 pound shelled edamame, blanched until tender-crisp

1 red onion, diced

1½ cups diced celery

2 red bell peppers, roasted (see note, page 26) and diced

2 yellow bell peppers, roasted (see note, page 26) and diced

2 green bell peppers, diced

2 avocados, diced

1 cup cooked corn kernels

1 cup coarsely chopped fresh cilantro

1 cup Basil Vinaigrette (page 40)

½ cup chopped Italian parsley

Combine all the ingredients in a large bowl and toss gently to avoid mashing the avocado. Serve in small bowls or on a bed of lettuce.

Edamame are green soybean pods. You're supposed to stick the pod into your mouth, bite down, and pull it back out, squishing out the delicious green soybeans (you eat the beans and discard the pods). The beans can usually be found in the frozen section of supermarkets and natural food stores, conveniently shelled. Soybeans are known to be high in protein, calcium, and cancer-fighting antioxidants. Not only that, they're good to eat! This salad has been a runaway hit every time I've served it.

Dilled Tomato Salad

Makes 4 servings

4 to 6 vine-ripened tomatoes, peeled, cut in half, and thinly sliced

½ small red onion, very thinly sliced

2 tablespoons chopped fresh dill

¼ cup Udo's Oil

2 tablespoons red wine vinegar

¼ teaspoon sea salt

¼ teaspoon freshly ground black pepper

Place the tomatoes in a bowl and cover them with the onion and dill. Place the oil, vinegar, salt, and pepper in a jar and shake well. Pour over the tomato mixture and toss gently to mix. Taste and adjust the seasonings, if needed. Serve at once.

There's nothing like a fresh-picked tomato, still warm from the sun, sliced up with nothing but salt and pepper on it. This salad is a pretty close second, adding a northern European influence with fresh dill and red wine vinegar.

If you prefer, serve this salad on a bed of sliced dandelion leaves. Mmmmm!

French Bean Salad

Makes 4 to 6 servings

1 pound green beans

1 medium red onion, finely diced

2 tablespoons chopped fresh parsley

1/2 cup or more PseUdo French Dressing (page 44), prepared with double the mustard

1/2 to 1 cup grated Parmesan cheese

Sea salt

Freshly ground black pepper

2 to 3 medium tomatoes, cut in half and sliced

12 kalamata or niçoise olives

*C*ut the green beans on a sharp diagonal, producing fairly long thin strips. Blanch them in salted water until just tender-crisp. Drain, plunge into ice water to stop the cooking completely, drain again, and spread on a towel to dry.

Combine the beans, onion, and half of the parsley in a large bowl. Add the dressing and 1/2 cup of the Parmesan cheese and stir well. Taste and add more dressing and cheese, if you like. Season with salt and pepper to taste, if needed.

Mound the mixture on an oval platter or in a large bowl. Surround it with the tomato slices, slightly overlapping them. Scatter the olives over the top and sprinkle with the remaining parsley. Serve at once, or cover and refrigerate until serving time.

The proper title of this recipe might have been Frenched Bean Salad, since these are regular green beans cut on a sharp diagonal, or "French cut," and not actually French beans (also known as *haricots verts*, or tiny tender baby green beans). And I would have called it that, but in high school the term "frenched" meant having gone a step beyond mere lip kissing, which I thought might sound weird in reference to the beans. Never mind—this is a fantastic salad (owed mostly, I suspect, to the presence of Parmesan cheese).

Fresh Artichokes with Mint

Makes 4 to 6 servings

2 cloves garlic
1 teaspoon sea salt
3 tablespoons freshly squeezed lemon juice
3 tablespoons Udo's Oil
8 large globe artichokes
1 lemon, cut in half
$1/4$ cup chopped fresh mint

*T*o make the dressing, put the garlic through a garlic press and mash the pulp with the back of a wooden spoon into a smooth purée. Work in the salt, then the lemon juice and the oil.

Snap off the outer leaves the artichokes; they should break fairly flush with the base. Peel away the dark outer flesh of the artichokes with a paring knife, and then use a spoon to pry out the hairy choke, leaving only the bottoms and the pale, tender parts of the leaves. If any bits of the choke remain, rinse them away under running water. Rub the artichokes with the lemon to prevent discoloration as you work. Slice the artichoke bottoms about $1/8$ inch thick and immediately stir them into the dressing. Add the mint and stir well. Let rest a few minutes before serving.

Most people have not tried artichokes other than the standard way—cooked whole and served with melted butter to dip the leaves into——let alone raw in a salad! This recipe may be a bit of a hassle to prepare, but it's well worth it.

Salads

Grated Fresh Beet Salad

Makes 4 servings

2 medium beets, peeled and grated

4 stalks celery, strings removed, cut in half lengthwise, and thinly sliced

1 red bell pepper, diced

12 radishes, diced

1 small carrot, grated

1/2 cup Sweet Balsamic Vinaigrette (page 54)

4 cups baby romaine leaves

2 tablespoons snipped chives

*T*oss the beets, celery, bell pepper, radishes, and carrot with the vinaigrette and let rest several minutes. Divide the lettuce leaves among four plates. Toss the salad again and place a mound on each bed of lettuce. Top with the snipped chives and serve at once.

Be sure to wear an apron and roll up your sleeves when you grate the beets. Once you've covered that step, the rest is a snap. Now you've got a brilliant salad. Go, eat, and be healthy!

Pungent Coleslaw

Makes 4 to 6 servings

2 cups red cabbage, thinly sliced

2 cups green cabbage, thinly sliced

1 cup red onion, thinly sliced

4 stalks celery, strings removed, cut in half lengthwise,
    and thinly sliced diagonally

2 carrots, shredded

8 scallions, sliced diagonally

2 tablespoons coarsely chopped fresh cilantro

3/4 cup Asian Miso Dressing (page 40)

*C*ombine all the vegetables in a large bowl. Cover and chill until ready to serve. Prepare the dressing at the last possible minute, add to the vegetables, toss thoroughly, and serve at once.

The secret to this salad is to make the dressing just before tossing it with the slaw and serve it right away. It's still pretty good even the next day, but the juices will have drained from the vegetables, and it won't be nearly as vibrant.

Greek Salad

8 cups mixed salad greens (such as romaine, red leaf, and endive)

1 to 2 medium red onions, sliced and separated into rings

1 cucumber, sliced

2 to 4 medium tomatoes, cut into wedges

1 green bell pepper, cut into strips

8 large radishes, sliced

2 to 3 stalks celery, strings removed and sliced

2 tablespoons chopped fresh dill

1/4 cup chopped fresh parsley

8 ounces feta cheese, cut into small cubes

1/2 to 3/4 cup kalamata olives

1 to 2 tablespoons capers

1/2 cup Fast Greek Salad Dressing (page 43)

*W*ash and spin the greens dry or roll them up gently in a towel and crisp them in the refrigerator while you prepare the rest of the salad. Put the greens in a large bowl. Arrange the other ingredients on top, in the order listed. Get everyone together. Shake the dressing, sprinkle it over the salad, and toss. Serve and eat. Sing, dance, break the dishes, fight, and so forth.

What follows is just a guideline. Use whichever ingredients you like, in whatever proportions you like, omitting whichever ones you don't like. Pretty much the only ingredients everyone agrees *must* be in a Greek salad are the feta, the olives, and (duh!) the greens. Some hard-core Grecophiles may insist on anchovies (the high cost of fanaticism), some may insist on tomato and cucumber, but actually the Greeks are pretty easygoing, so as long as the feta, olives, and greens are there, you've got yourself a Greek salad.

Hot-and-Sour Potato Salad

Makes 4 to 6 servings

1½ pounds new potatoes, scrubbed well

1 tablespoon plus ½ teaspoon sea salt

1 Maui onion (see note), cut in half and thinly sliced

1 bunch scallions, sliced diagonally

½ cup chopped fresh cilantro

4 cloves garlic, peeled and minced

1 or 2 hot green chiles, finely chopped

¼ cup Udo's Oil

3 tablespoons soy sauce

1 tablespoon freshly squeezed lime juice

1 tablespoon Sriracha Sauce (page 38)

1 tablespoon tamarind paste (see note, page 33)

½ teaspoon freshly ground black pepper

*B*ring about 2 quarts of water to a boil. Add the potatoes and 1 tablespoon of the salt. Return to a boil, reduce the heat to medium, and cook for 15 to 20 minutes, or until the potatoes are just tender. Drain and refresh under cold water. Cut the potatoes in half.

While the potatoes are cooking, combine the onion, scallions, cilantro, garlic, and chiles in a large bowl. Combine the oil, soy sauce, lime juice, Sriracha Sauce, tamarind paste, the remaining ½ teaspoon salt, and the pepper in a small bowl and stir into the onion mixture. Add the potatoes while they're still warm and toss gently but thoroughly. Let rest for about 10 minutes, then taste the potatoes and adjust the seasonings, if needed. Serve at room temperature—on a banana leaf, if any are available!

It's good to have more than a couple of ways to make a potato salad, and this one is really different—better than any other I know. If you ever saw the film *The Year of Living Dangerously*, this salad would fit right in. "You're in old Java now, boss."

Maui onions are sweet and mild. If you can't find any where you live, try Vidalia, which are similar, or as a last resort, red onion.

Mediterranean Roasted Vegetable Salad

Makes 6 to 8 servings

3 ripe tomatoes

3 eggplants

2 red onions

$1/3$ cup extra-virgin olive oil

2 red bell peppers, roasted (see note, page 26)
and cut into $1/2$-inch strips

$1/2$ cup chopped Italian parsley

$2/3$ cup Udo's Oil

$1/2$ cup freshly squeezed lemon juice

3 cloves garlic, peeled and minced

1 teaspoon sea salt

$1/2$ teaspoon freshly ground black pepper

On a hot summer day this salad and some crusty bread are all you'll really need for lunch. It also makes a terrific buffet item.

Preheat the oven to 400 degrees F and line a baking sheet with parchment paper. Rub the tomatoes, eggplants, and onions with a little of the olive oil and place them on the prepared baking sheet. Prick the eggplant in several places with a fork. Roast the vegetables for 15 minutes, until the tomato skins begin to blister. Remove the tomatoes and continue roasting the onions and eggplants until they are tender, about 1 hour longer. Set aside to cool. Peel the vegetables. Slice the onions about $1/2$ inch thick. Tear the eggplants into thick strips. Cut the tomatoes into $3/4$-inch cubes. Combine with the peppers and parsley in a large bowl.

Whisk together the Udo's Oil, lemon juice, the remaining olive oil, and the garlic, salt, and pepper until well emulsified. Pour over the vegetables and toss well. Taste and adjust the seasonings, if needed. Serve at once.

Mexican Potato Salad

Makes 6 to 8 servings

- 3 pounds russet potatoes
- 2 white or red onions, finely diced
- 1 cup Udo's Oil
- 1 cup chopped fresh cilantro
- $1/2$ cup red wine vinegar
- 4 serrano chiles, finely diced (optional)
- $1^1/2$ teaspoons sea salt
- $1/2$ teaspoon freshly ground black pepper

Cook the potatoes in boiling salted water until just barely tender. While the potatoes are cooking, combine the remaining ingredients in a large bowl. When the potatoes are done, drain and refresh them in cold water until just cool enough to handle. Peel the potatoes and cut them into $3/4$-inch dice. Add the warm potatoes to the rest of the salad and toss well. Serve this on lettuce leaves, in bowls, or in a large dish as part of a summer buffet.

In Mexico this goes by the unexciting name *ensalada de papa* (potato salad), belying the dazzling, pungent tastes that explode in your mouth as you eat it. Very quick and easy to prepare, it's a tasty alternative to the ubiquitous American heavy-mayo potato salad.

Portobello Mushroom Salad

Makes 4 servings

1 tablespoon extra-virgin olive oil

$1/4$ cup red wine

2 cloves garlic, peeled, crushed, and minced

1 bay leaf

4 portobello mushrooms, washed and stems gently pried out

$1/2$ teaspoon sea salt

$1/2$ teaspoon freshly ground black pepper

$1/2$ cup Udo's Oil

$1/4$ cup aged balsamic vinegar (see note, page 111)

4 shallots, finely diced

2 tablespoons snipped chives

2 tablespoons chopped fresh parsley

Originally, when I came up with this salad, I used to rub olive oil and garlic over the mushrooms and then grill them. The result was a charred exterior with a tender interior. Udo has since straightened me out on the grilling part, so here's the new version. It's good served by itself in a bowl or with tender greens like mâche or frisée.

Spread the olive oil in a large skillet and add the wine, garlic, and bay leaf. Heat gently, stirring until the mixture bubbles. Season the mushroom caps on both sides with half of the salt and pepper and place them in the skillet, cap side down. Cover tightly and raise the heat to high. As soon as the mushrooms begin to release their juices into the simmering liquid in the pan, lower the heat and cook for about 5 minutes. Remove the lid, turn the mushrooms over, and cook uncovered until the liquid is absorbed. Remove the skillet from the heat and allow the mushrooms to cool. Slice them thinly.

Whisk the Udo's Oil, vinegar, and remaining salt and pepper in a large bowl. When the dressing emulsifies, whisk in the shallots. Add the sliced mushrooms and toss well. Combine the chives and parsley in a small bowl. Reserve 1 tablespoon for garnish, add the rest to the mushroom mixture, and toss well. Pile the salad in a serving dish and sprinkle the reserved herbs on top. Serve at once.

Roasted Beet Salad

Makes 6 to 8 servings

- 2 pounds beets, well scrubbed
- 1 tablespoon chopped fresh thyme
- 2 tablespoons extra-virgin olive oil
- 4 cloves garlic, pressed or peeled and minced
- 1 teaspoon sea salt
- $1/2$ teaspoon freshly ground black pepper
- 1 bunch celery
- 2 fennel bulbs, cored and finely diced
- 1 red onion, finely diced
- 1 cup Roasted Garlic Vinaigrette (page 48)
- Arugula (optional)

*P*reheat the oven to 375 degrees F. Cut the beets into quarters. If they vary in size, cut the smaller ones in half so all the pieces are uniform. Combine the thyme, olive oil, garlic, salt, and pepper. Mix well and toss with the beets. Transfer to a heavy baking dish, cover with foil, and roast for about 1 hour, or until the beets are fork-tender. Let cool with the cover in place.

While the beets are cooking, separate the celery stalks. Remove and set aside the tender inner leaves for garnish. Remove the strings from the celery and cut the celery into fine dice. Cut the beets into $1/2$-inch dice and toss them with the celery, fennel, and onion. Add the dressing and toss again. Let rest for about 10 minutes to allow the flavors to develop, then taste and adjust the seasonings, if needed. Serve in bowls or on plates over a bed of arugula, if desired. Garnish with the reserved celery leaves.

Just the smell of fresh thyme filling the kitchen is worth the effort to make this salad, believe me. Plus, this is a mighty fine dish. If you like goat cheese, add a generous slice to the plate—it goes superbly with this salad.

Photo: Poached Eggs with Avocado and Chipotle Sauce (page 80), black beans and Oily Salsa (page 72)

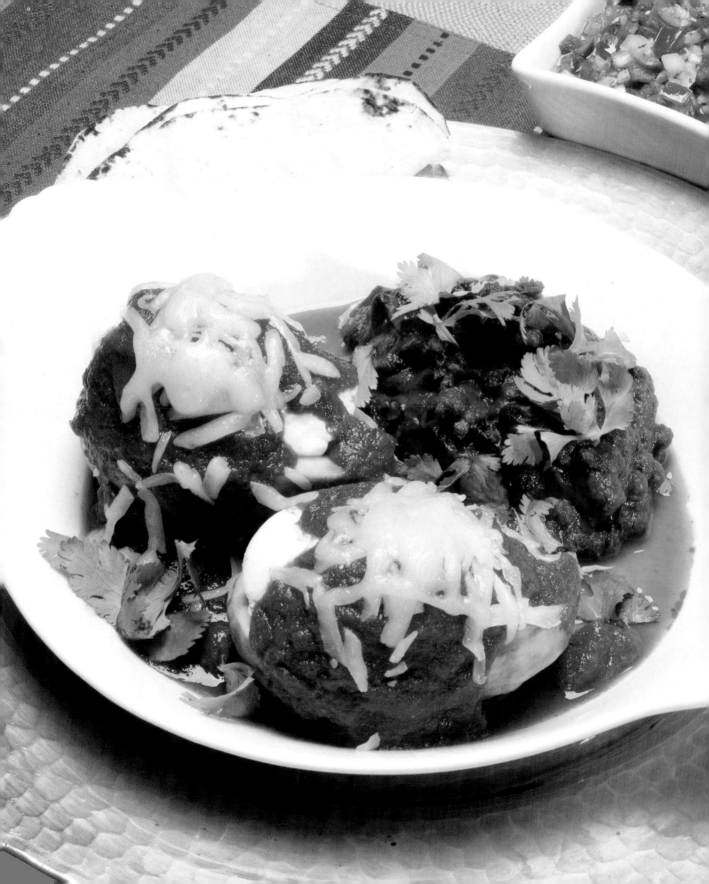

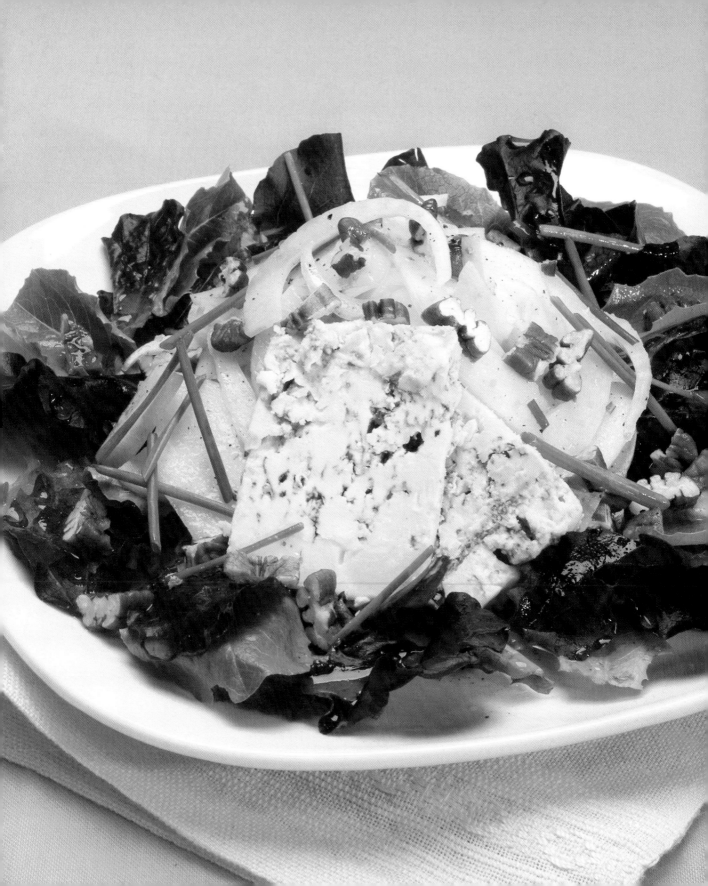

Tomato Salad
with Basil Oil

Makes 4 servings

4 to 6 vine-ripened tomatoes, peeled and thickly sliced
1 clove garlic, peeled and minced
½ small red onion, thinly sliced
¼ cup Basil Oil (page 22)
¼ teaspoon sea salt
¼ teaspoon freshly ground black pepper
1 tablespoon finely chopped fresh parsley

*A*rrange the tomato slices in a circle on individual serving plates, slightly overlapping them. Strew the garlic and onion over the tomatoes and drizzle liberally with the Basil Oil. Season with the salt and pepper, and sprinkle the parsley on top. Serve at once.

> If you prefer, serve the salad on a bed of watercress or arugula. If the tomatoes are really spectacular, you might want to omit the garlic and onion and celebrate just the tomato itself, using only the Basil Oil, salt, and pepper to set it off. Your call.

Once nature has done its thing, creating beautiful, juicy, perfect red tomatoes, the job's nearly done. They should have just enough acidity to balance the oil, with no need for any vinegar. This salad is at its absolute best when the tomatoes are fresh off the vine, still warm, with that unmistakable just-picked-from-the-field taste.

Photo: Apple and Fennel Salad with Saint Agūr (page 110)

Tabouli

1 cup seeded and finely diced cucumber

1 cup bulgur (see note)

2 cups chopped fresh parsley

1 cup chopped fresh mint

1 cup chopped scallions

1 cup chopped tomatoes

4 or more cloves garlic, peeled and minced

1/2 cup freshly squeezed lemon juice

1/4 cup Udo's Oil

1/4 cup extra-virgin olive oil

1 teaspoon sea salt

1/2 teaspoon freshly ground black pepper

*L*ightly salt the cucumber and set aside. Cover the bulgur with boiling water and let rest for 20 minutes. Drain the bulgur, gently squeeze out the excess water, put it into a large bowl, and fluff it to help it cool completely. Drain the cucumber and add it to the bulgur along with the parsley, mint, scallions, tomatoes, and garlic. Mix well. Whisk together the lemon juice, Udo's Oil, olive oil, salt, and pepper and add it to the bulgur and vegetables. Stir well and let rest for at least 15 minutes to allow the flavors to develop.

Tabouli is best served at room temperature, right after it's made, when all the pungent qualities of the vegetables are at their peak of exploding freshness. If it must wait longer than an hour or two, cover and refrigerate. Remove from the refrigerator and uncover about 20 minutes before serving. Any leftovers can be saved for a day or two and will still be quite delicious, although the original spark will have gone out.

The secret to good tabouli is in the proportion of parsley and mint to bulgur. It should be very green with little flecks of white, not the other way around. Think salad, not grain, and you'll do fine. You might try experimenting with the ratio of olive oil to Udo's Oil, maximizing on the latter as much as possible. Also—and this is heresy—try substituting cooked quinoa (see note, page 79) for the bulgur. I discovered this because my son has a wheat allergy, and the rest of us wanted some tabouli. Quinoa is high in protein and quite delicious; in tabouli, it's even better than bulgur (in my opinion, of course). Try it both ways and decide for yourself.

Bulgur is made from whole wheat berries that have been parboiled, dried, and crushed. It is reconstituted by soaking in hot water or broth and requires no cooking. Featured in Middle Eastern cuisine, bulgur is higher in protein than rice or couscous. Look for it at natural food stores and well-stocked supermarkets.

Salad of Flageolets
with Tarragon Vinaigrette

Makes 6 to 8 servings

3/4 pound flageolets (see note)

1 bay leaf

1 large carrot, finely diced and blanched until tender-crisp

1 cup finely diced celery

1 cup finely diced fennel

1 yellow bell pepper, roasted (see note, page 26) and finely diced

1 green bell pepper, roasted (see note, page 26) and finely diced

1/2 cup chopped Italian parsley

4 shallots, finely diced

1 avocado, diced

1 cup Tarragon Vinaigrette (page 50)

Heirloom tomato slices (see note)

1/2 cup tender celery leaves

1/4 cup snipped chives

Pick over the beans, removing any stones or other debris, and wash in cold water. Place in a pot and cover with cold water by about 4 inches. Add the bay leaf and bring to a boil. Lower the heat to maintain a steady simmer and cook for 20 to 45 minutes, or until just tender (the cooking time will depend on the age of the beans). When the beans are almost tender, add the salt and stir well. When the beans are done, remove from the heat and let cool completely. Drain well.

Toss the beans with the carrot, celery, fennel, peppers, parsley, and shallots. Add the avocado and dressing and toss again gently to avoid mashing the avocado. Arrange a few tomato slices on salad plates, mound the salad in the center, and garnish with the celery leaves and chives.

For some reason flageolets and tarragon just go together, don't ask me why. Served on slices of heirloom tomatoes, this salad is as close to perfection as beans, or tarragon, will ever get.

Flageolets are a type of dried bean with a pale green color. They are favored in France for their unique flavor and creamy texture and can be found in most specialty stores and in the gourmet section of some supermarkets.

Heirloom tomatoes are unparalleled for their taste, texture, and unique appearance. Look for them at farmer's markets and some specialty grocery stores. However, do not by any means pass on this recipe if you can't find them. Any high-quality, ripe tomato will do just fine.

Udo's Caesar Salad

Makes 4 servings

- 2 medium heads romaine lettuce
- 4 thick slices French bread
- 1/4 cup Simple Garlic Oil (page 22)
- 1/3 cup freshly squeezed lemon juice
- 1 egg yolk
- 4 cloves garlic, peeled
- 1/2 teaspoon sea salt
- 1/2 teaspoon freshly ground black pepper
- 2/3 cup Udo's Oil
- 1 1/4 cups freshly grated Parmigiano-Reggiano

*W*ash and tear the lettuce into large bite-size pieces. Keep refrigerated until ready to assemble the salad.

Preheat the oven to 275 degrees F. Place the bread slices on a baking sheet and bake until fairly crisp, 10 to 20 minutes. Brush generously with the Simple Garlic Oil and carefully cut into croutons with a serrated knife. Leave uncovered at room temperature; they will crisp further as they cool.

For the dressing, combine the lemon juice, egg yolk, garlic, salt, and pepper in a blender and process until smooth. With the motor running, slowly pour in the Udo's Oil. Add 1/2 cup of the cheese and pulse until blended. Pour into a small container and stir in another 1/2 cup of the cheese by hand. Refrigerate until ready to use.

To serve, toss the salad in a large bowl with a small amount of the dressing. Taste and add more dressing, if needed. Refrigerate any leftover dressing in an airtight jar for up to 1 week. Add the croutons and toss again. Divide among four plates, sprinkle the remaining cheese on top, and serve immediately.

Not too many people know this, but Caesar salad was not invented in Italy or named for Emperor Julius. It was invented by Cesar Cardini, at his Italian restaurant in, of all places, Tijuana, Mexico. An argument has been made that this is actually a Mexican dish. The original salad had whole romaine leaves, tossed tableside with the other ingredients added one by one. Large crostini, made from Mexican *bolillos* and smeared with anchovy paste, were added last.

In my version, no one is ever going to know you've substituted Udo's Oil for the usual olive oil. The dressing is perfect, owing in no small part to the use of genuine imported Parmigiano-Reggiano, which, let's face it, is the only real Parmesan cheese there is (accept no substitutes!). Also, if you're serving any nonvegetarians, just don't mention the absence of anchovies, and the subject won't even come up. Vegans, sadly, will have to sit this one out.

Don't be afraid of the raw egg yolk. The acid in the lemon juice will kill any microscopic creeps lurking about. (See note, page 185.)

Beans and Grains

While it's possible to enjoy beans and grains alone, it's the addition of vegetables (and fats) that make them especially palatable. Most Americans plan their menu around one slab of meat or another, with everything else on the plate considered an optional garnish. Vegetarians, on the other hand, regard every item on the plate equally, each with its own special flavors and qualities. Beans and grains, whether combined in one dish or kept separate, share equal importance with vegetables. This, in my opinion, is the way it should be, even for those who consider meat or fish an essential part of their diet.

The recipes in this section, as in the section on vegetables, should help anyone who is new to a vegetarian diet and still somewhat stuck on the old meat-centered paradigm begin the transition to a more diverse approach. You'll find many ways to incorporate different sources of plant protein into your diet and enjoy new flavor sensations without having to resort to options that mimic meat. I've never been a fan of imitation meat, near-beer, or anything like that. The way I see it, if you're going to leave something behind, don't bring it with you.

Adzuki Beans with Deadly Nightshades

Makes 6 to 8 servings

1 pound dried adzuki beans

1 red onion, finely diced

1 green bell pepper, finely diced

1 cup peeled, seeded, and chopped tomatoes

1 tablespoon herbes de Provence

1 bay leaf

1 teaspoon sea salt

2 tablespoons chopped sun-dried tomatoes
   packed in extra-virgin olive oil

1 tablespoon chopped fresh parsley

1 tablespoon chopped fresh basil

½ cup Simple Garlic Oil (page 22)

*P*ick over the beans to remove any small stones or other debris. Wash well, drain, and place in a bowl with enough fresh water to cover by about 3 inches. Soak for 8 to 12 hours.

Drain the beans and place them in a heavy soup pot along with the onion, bell pepper, fresh tomatoes, herbes de Provence, and bay leaf. Add enough cold water to cover by about 2 inches and bring to a boil over medium-high heat. Lower the heat and simmer for about 1 hour, or until the beans are tender but still hold their shape. Add the salt and sun-dried tomatoes and cook for 5 to 10 minutes longer. The liquid should be fairly thick. Discard the bay leaf and stir in the parsley and basil. Remove from the heat and stir in the Simple Garlic Oil. Serve at once in bowls as a side dish or on a plate with rice and vegetables.

This is a joke, actually.
Adzuki beans are a favorite staple of those who follow a macrobiotic diet and shun peppers and tomatoes as members of the belladonna, or "deadly nightshade," family, which also includes eggplants and potatoes. Personally, I find it hard to imagine a decent cuisine utterly devoid of the nightshade crowd. This recipe takes adzuki beans on a vacation from their Asian roots for a sort of Mediterranean cruise. "Belladonna," by the way, is Italian for "beautiful woman," which is not a bad way to go, if you ask me.

Barley and Beets

Makes 4 to 6 servings

1 cup pearl barley

3 cups grated beets

2 cups vegetable broth or water

1 cup apple juice

1 medium red onion, finely diced

$1/2$ cup finely diced leek greens

$1/2$ cup diced celery

1 teaspoon sea salt

1 tablespoon aged balsamic vinegar (see note, page 111)

$1/2$ teaspoon freshly ground black pepper

2 bunches scallions, sliced

$1/2$ cup Udo's Oil

The sweetness and brilliant ruby red color of this dish lend barley a new life, especially for people who have only known it in a soup with mushrooms. It goes very nicely with other dishes, but stands quite well on its own. If you have any left over, serve it cold, with chopped fresh celery, scallions, parsley, and a touch more balsamic vinegar or lemon juice added, on a bed of lettuce.

*R*inse the barley well and drain. Place in a deep saucepan with the beets, broth, apple juice, onion, leek, celery, and salt. Bring to a boil. Reduce the heat to low, cover, and cook for 1 hour, or until all the liquid has been absorbed. After about 30 minutes, begin checking occasionally, stirring with a heat-proof rubber spatula or wooden spoon to prevent the mixture from sticking.

When the barley is tender and all the liquid has been absorbed, add the balsamic vinegar and the pepper. Taste and add more salt, if needed. Remove from the heat. Set aside a few tablespoons of the scallions for a garnish. Add the remaining scallions and the oil and stir well. Serve at once, garnished with the reserved scallions.

Bhutanese Red Rice Pilaf

Makes 4 to 6 servings

1 cup Bhutanese red rice

2 tablespoons extra-virgin olive oil

2 cups vegetable broth

1/2 cup fresh beet juice (see note)

1 teaspoon sea salt

1/4 teaspoon freshly ground black pepper

2 bunches scallions, sliced

1 cup chopped fresh cilantro

1/2 cup raw cashews

1/3 cup Simple Garlic Oil (page 22)

Wash the rice in cold water and drain. Spread out on a towel and rub to dry the grains. Pour the rice into a bowl, add the olive oil, and rub the rice between your hands to coat the grains evenly. Put the rice into a large pot with the broth, beet juice, salt, and pepper. Bring to a boil over high heat, reduce the heat to maintain a simmer, and cover the pot. Cook for 20 to 25 minutes, or until the grains are tender. Turn off the heat and stir in the scallions, cilantro, cashews, and Simple Garlic Oil. Taste and adjust the seasonings, if needed. Serve at once.

If you have a vegetable juicer, make the beet juice fresh. If not, you can buy it from your local juice bar. If neither of these options is available to you, substitute an equal amount of vegetable broth and proceed with the recipe. The color will not be as bright, but the Bhutanese don't use beet juice in their rice either, so you'll be in good company.

Bhutanese Red Rice

In case you haven't come across this unique rice, it is a staple in Bhutan, as well as in some neighboring Himalayan countries. It has a natural nutty flavor and a pleasant rust color when cooked. In my recipe, the color is heightened by the addition of beet juice. You can find Bhutanese red rice in Asian grocery stores, natural food stores, gourmet shops, and well-stocked supermarkets in the Asian section.

Black Beans
with Leek Greens and Hominy

Makes 6 servings

4 cups diced leek greens (tender green part only)

1 cup diced celery

1 cup diced white or Maui onion

1 tablespoon ghee (clarified butter) or extra-virgin olive oil

1 teaspoon sea salt

2½ cups vegetable broth

3 cups hominy

3 cups cooked black beans

1 large tomato, grated (about ½ cup)

2 tablespoons ancho chili powder

1 teaspoon piment d'Espelette (optional, but highly
    recommended; see note)

½ cup chopped fresh cilantro

¼ cup Simple Garlic Oil (page 22)

Combine the leeks, celery, onion, and ghee in a heavy saucepan and place over high heat, stirring constantly. As soon as you hear the first hint of sizzling, add the salt and 1 tablespoon of the broth. Continue stirring as the vegetables wilt slightly and slowly release their juices. When the vegetables are soft and almost no liquid remains in the bottom of the pan, add the remaining broth and the hominy, black beans, tomato, ancho chili powder, and optional piment d'Espelette. Bring to a boil, adjust the heat to maintain a steady simmer, and cook for about 20 minutes, or until everything is tender and the liquid is reduced to a sauce.

Remove from the heat and stir in the cilantro and Simple Garlic Oil. Serve in bowls.

This dish is a kind of stew made with black beans and hominy, which together make up a whole protein.

Hominy is white corn that has been treated with limewater, resulting in a grain with a unique flavor and more absorbable nutrients, including niacin, calcium, and amino acids. Called *nixtamal* in Mexico, it's used to make tortillas, tamales, and various regional dishes, including pozole.

Piment d'Espelette is a unique, sweet-hot pepper grown in just a few small villages in France. It is essential to authentic Basque cuisine. Piment d'Espelette is available in jars, dried and ground. If you cannot find the real thing, substitute Hungarian hot paprika, available in most supermarkets.

Brown Basmati Rice
with Burdock and Lotus Root

Makes 4 to 6 servings

4 small to medium burdock roots, well scrubbed (see note)

½ cup sake

½ cup soy sauce

½ cup mirin (see note)

¼ cup brown rice syrup (see note)

1 medium fresh lotus root (see note), peeled
   and very thinly sliced

1 cup brown basmati rice

2 cups vegetable broth

1 bunch scallions, sliced

⅓ cup Simple Garlic Oil (page 22)

*L*ay one of the burdock roots on a cutting board and trim the root end on a diagonal. Roll the burdock root toward you about one-quarter turn and cut it on the diagonal. Roll it another quarter turn and cut again. Repeat this process all the way to the end, then follow the same process with the other burdock roots. You should have interesting shapes, each with one round side and a couple of flat sides. This is called the Chinese rolling cut (cool, huh?).

Combine the sake, soy sauce, mirin, and brown rice syrup in a deep saucepan. Add the burdock and lotus root, place over high heat, and bring to a boil. Adjust the heat to maintain a low simmer, cover, and cook slowly until the vegetables are tender, about 1 hour or longer. These vegetables will retain an assertive little crunch even after they're done, so just use your judgment on this. If the sauce gets too thick, add a little water from time to time.

With an atypical combination of textures and flavors, this dish is downright delicious. Even fast-food-addicted kids will eat this. The slices of lotus root give it an exotic visual effect with their unusual shape, which is new to most Westerners. Ask for fresh lotus root and burdock root at Asian grocers and most well-stocked natural food stores. Sometimes they may have to order it for you, but it's worth the wait.

While the vegetables are cooking, rinse the rice in cold water and drain. Put it in a large pot with the broth and bring to a boil over high heat. Reduce the heat to maintain a simmer and cover the pot. Cook until the grains are tender, 45 minutes to 1 hour.

As soon as both vegetables and rice are done, remove them from the heat; toss them together, and stir in the scallions and Simple Garlic Oil. Serve at once.

Burdock root is a fibrous vegetable with a sweet, earthy taste; it is favored by those who practice macrobiotics. In Chinese medicine it is considered a strong blood purifier. Look for it in natural food stores and Asian markets, where it is known by its Japanese name, gobo. Depending on freshness, the dark skin may come off when scrubbed, or it may remain intact. Either way, the vegetable is delicious.

Brown rice syrup is a gentle, delicate sweetener.

Mirin is a sweet Japanese cooking wine. Along with mirin (above), it can be found in Asian grocery stores and natural food stores.

Lotus root is an extremely nutritious food, rich in vitamin C, potassium, thiamin, riboflavin, vitamin B_6, phosphorus, copper, and manganese. It is also high in dietary fiber. The skin is very tough and must be removed. A vegetable peeler works well for this, but several passes may be required to reach the lighter-colored, relatively tender flesh underneath.

Dal Saag

Makes 4 to 6 servings

1 cup dried moong dal (skinned)

4 cups water

1 small tomato, grated

7 cloves garlic, peeled and minced

2 green chiles, chopped or sliced

2 tablespoons peeled and minced ginger

1 tablespoon ground coriander

1 teaspoon ground cumin

$1/2$ teaspoon cayenne

$1/4$ teaspoon turmeric

$1/4$ teaspoon asafetida (see note)

1 pound fresh spinach, chopped

1 bunch scallions, chopped

$1^1/2$ teaspoons sea salt

$1/2$ cup Udo's Oil

*P*ick over the dal to remove any small stones or other debris. Wash well. Bring the water to a boil in a heavy pot and add the dal. Return to a boil and cook uncovered for about 5 minutes, skimming the foam frequently. Add the tomato, garlic, green chiles, ginger, coriander, cumin, cayenne, turmeric, and asafetida. Return to a boil, lower the heat to maintain a slow, steady simmer, cover, and cook until the dal is soft, about 40 minutes or longer. Check often during the last 10 minutes and stir frequently to prevent sticking. Add a little more boiling water, if needed.

When the dal is tender, raise the heat to high and stir in the spinach, scallions, and salt. Cook just until the greens are tender—no longer than 2 to 3 minutes.

Remove from the heat and stir in the oil. Serve at once, in bowls as a side dish or with rice and vegetables.

In Indian cooking, dal (see below) is made by first cooking the beans or lentils and then quickly frying the aromatics and adding them toward the end. In this heretical version, the aromatics are cooked into the beans without frying, and the oil is added after the cooking is done. It tastes pretty darn good anyway—and it might even fool some of your Indian friends. There are two kinds of *moong dal*, with and without their green skin. For this dish, buy the skinned ones, which look a little bit like small, ivory-colored barley.

Dal is the Hindi word for pulses (lentils and beans), as well as any of the numerous Indian dishes that include them. Vastly varied in its forms and preparations throughout India, dal is virtually the sole sustenance for millions of people, often supplemented only with the homemade whole wheat flatbreads, *chapatis.*

Asafetida is the hardened sap of a variety of fennel cultivated in Asia. Called *hing* in Hindi, it is used in Indian cuisine, especially in lentil dishes, both for flavor and as a digestive aid. It has a very strong odor, which mellows during cooking. As the resin is rock hard, most people prefer to buy it preground. Asafetida is available in Indian grocery stores, natural food stores, and specialty markets.

Fassolada

Makes 6 to 8 servings

1 pound dried cannellini beans

4 stalks celery, with leaves, strings removed and diced

4 very thin carrots, sliced

1 large onion, finely diced

1 tablespoon minced garlic

1 tablespoon sea salt

1/2 cup Simple Garlic Oil (page 22)

1/4 cup coarsely chopped fresh parsley

2 tablespoons extra-virgin olive oil

6 to 12 slices feta cheese

Back when the Greeks conquered the world, this classic peasant dish was one of their staples. Brilliantly simple, this is about as satisfying as food gets. I suspect that something about the smell of beans cooking sets you up for it. Makes you want to dance around on ancient flagstones, make love, search for Truth, carve statues, and all that passionate stuff. *Eudaimonia!*

*P*ick over the beans to remove any small stones or other debris. Wash well, drain, place in a heavy soup pot, and add enough water to cover by about 3 inches. Bring to a boil, remove from the heat, and allow the beans soak at room temperature for about 2 hours.

Add the celery, carrots, onion, garlic, and enough water to cover by about 2 inches. Bring to a boil, lower the heat to maintain a steady simmer, and cook for 25 minutes or longer, until the beans are tender but still hold their shape.

Once the beans are tender, add the salt and cook very gently for 5 to 10 minutes longer. The liquid should be slightly soupy. Remove from the heat and stir in the Simple Garlic Oil, parsley, and olive oil. Ladle into wide soup bowls and serve at once, with the feta cheese on the side. Some crusty bread would be good with this, too.

Black Rice with Bok Choy

Makes 4 to 6 servings

1 cup black rice (see note)

2 cups vegetable broth

1/2 red onion, finely diced

1/2 teaspoon sea salt

1/4 cup sake

3 tablespoons soy sauce

3 tablespoons mirin (see note, page 139)

1 to 2 tablespoons peeled and grated fresh ginger

1 teaspoon Sriracha Sauce (page 38; optional)

2 tablespoons freshly squeezed lime juice

1 large bunch bok choy, coarsely chopped

2 bunches scallions, sliced diagonally

1/2 cup Simple Garlic Oil (page 22)

2 tablespoons chopped fresh cilantro

Black rice makes for a dramatic presentation with anything, but it's especially suited for the taste, texture, and color contrasts in this dish, combining the earthiness of the rice with the rich, bright notes from Asian seasonings, scallions, and bok choy. It's almost a one-dish meal.

*W*ash the rice well, drain, and place it in a bowl with enough fresh water to cover by about 1 inch. Let soak for about 1 hour. Drain and place in a heavy saucepan with the broth, onion, and salt. Bring to a boil, reduce the heat to low, and stir to mix well. Cover and cook for about 35 minutes, or until the liquid has been absorbed and the grains are tender. Cover and keep warm in a very low oven (around 250 degrees F) until serving time. This should be no more than 30 minutes; if you want to prepare the rice in advance, allow it to cool, refrigerate it, and then reheat it in a low oven until warmed through.

Combine the sake, soy sauce, mirin, ginger, and optional Sriracha Sauce in a small bowl. Keep the lime juice separate, in a small dish. Have a large pot of boiling salted water ready.

Just before serving, blanch the bok choy in the boiling salted water for about 45 seconds. Immediately drain in a large colander and return to the pot. Quickly add all the other ingredients, including the rice, sake mixture, and lime juice, and toss well. Serve at once.

Black rice— also known as black japonica, China black, and forbidden rice—is a whole grain, high in fiber and iron, with a delicious nutty flavor and a dark purple-black color when cooked. In Chinese medicine, it is considered a blood tonifier. Look for it in specialty shops and natural food stores.

Lentils with Swiss Chard

Makes 6 to 8 servings

12 ounces large dried green lentils

1 large onion, finely diced

2 tablespoons minced garlic

1 teaspoon ground cumin

1 teaspoon ground coriander

1 teaspoon hot paprika

1 teaspoon cayenne

½ teaspoon freshly ground black pepper

1 pound Swiss chard leaves, ribs removed and coarsely chopped

1 cup finely chopped fresh cilantro

1 teaspoon sea salt

3 tablespoons Udo's Oil

2 tablespoons extra-virgin olive oil

1 tablespoon freshly squeezed lemon juice

In Middle Eastern cooking, lentils and greens are a recurring combination. This one is a twenty-year favorite of mine. The trick is to cook the greens just long enough to make them tender, but not so long as to render them mushy and tasteless.

*P*ick over the lentils to remove any small stones or other debris. Wash well and place in a heavy soup pot. Add enough cold water to cover by about 1 inch and bring to a boil over medium-high heat. Add the onion, garlic, cumin, coriander, paprika, cayenne, and pepper. Adjust the heat to maintain a steady simmer and cook for 15 minutes.

Stir in the Swiss chard and cilantro. Cook for 5 to 10 minutes, or until the lentils are tender and the liquid is reduced to a sauce. Add the salt and cook for 1 to 2 minutes longer. Taste and add more salt, if needed. Remove from the heat and stir in the Udo's Oil, olive oil, and lemon juice. Serve at once.

Masoor Dal with Fenugreek

Makes 4 to 6 servings

1 cup dried masoor dal

4$\frac{1}{2}$ to 6 cups water

1 teaspoon sea salt

$\frac{1}{2}$ red onion, chopped

1 Roma tomato, chopped

2 tablespoons peeled and minced fresh ginger

7 cloves garlic, peeled

1$\frac{1}{2}$ teaspoons ground coriander

$\frac{1}{2}$ teaspoon turmeric

$\frac{1}{4}$ teaspoon ground cumin

$\frac{1}{4}$ teaspoon cayenne

3 bunches fresh fenugreek (see note, page 115)

$\frac{1}{2}$ cup Simple Garlic Oil (page 22)

*P*ick over the dal to remove any small stones or other debris. Wash well. Bring 4 cups of the water and the salt to a boil in a heavy pot and add the dal. Return to a boil and cook uncovered for about 5 minutes. Meanwhile, combine the onion, tomato, ginger, garlic, coriander, turmeric, cumin, and cayenne in a blender and process until smooth. Add to the pot, rinse the blender out with about $\frac{1}{2}$ cup of the remaining water, and add this to the pot as well. Return to a boil. Reduce the heat to low, cover, and cook for about 20 minutes, or until very soft. Stir every few minutes toward the end to prevent the dal from sticking.

While the dal is cooking, wash the fenugreek thoroughly and remove any tough stems. Chop the leaves and tender stems coarsely. Once the dal is soft (the mixture will be fairly thick and mushy at this point), stir in the fenugreek. This should thin the mixture down a bit, but if it is still too dry, add a little more water. Continue cooking for 3 to 5 minutes longer, or until the fenugreek is tender. Remove from the heat and stir in the Simple Garlic Oil. Serve at once, in bowls as a side dish or on a plate with rice and vegetables.

This is blasphemy. In Indian cooking, *dal* is generally prepared by first boiling the lentils or beans, and aromatics fried in oil or clarified butter are added near the end. Of course, in this book we never fry anything (especially never in Udo's Oil!). For recreating a similarly gratifying dish without frying, the following recipe works well. Look for *masoor dal*, a bright orange split lentil, at Indian grocery stores and natural food stores.

Mung Beans
with Ginger and Garlic

Makes 6 to 8 servings

1 pound dried whole mung beans (with skin)

1 large red onion, finely diced

6 tablespoons peeled and minced fresh ginger

1/4 cup minced garlic

2 tablespoons garam masala (see note)

2 tablespoons ground coriander

2 teaspoons turmeric

1 tablespoon sea salt

1 to 2 bunches cilantro, coarsely chopped

1 cup Simple Garlic Oil (page 22)

*P*ick over the beans to remove any small stones or other debris. Wash well, drain, and place in a heavy soup pot along with the onion, ginger, garlic, garam masala, coriander, and turmeric. Add enough cold water to cover by about 2 inches and bring to a boil over medium-high heat. Adjust the heat to maintain a steady simmer and cook for 45 to 60 minutes, or until the beans are tender but still hold their shape. Add the salt and cook for 5 to 10 minutes longer. The liquid should be fairly thick; if not, cook a little longer. Stir in the cilantro. Remove from the heat and stir in the Simple Garlic Oil. Serve at once, in bowls as a side dish or on a plate with rice and vegetables.

Each time I prepare a dish like this, it feels like another stake is driven into the heart of authentic Indian food. But the greatness of that kingly cuisine somehow manages to shine through, even if the method is jumbled, the ingredients are tampered with, or the cook is not Indian. The gods are tolerant, what can I tell you?

Garam masala, a mixture of ground spices used in Indian cuisine, varies widely, depending on the region as well as the cook. The name means "hot spice," although chiles are not always included; the "heat" also comes from pungent ingredients such as cassia bark, cardamom, cinnamon, and cloves. Indian cooks freshly grind their own preferred mixtures to get the most vibrant flavor and aroma, since ground spices lose quite a bit of their potency over time. Most Western cooks prefer to buy commercial garam masala for convenience. Look for it in Indian grocery stores, natural food stores, gourmet shops, and well-stocked supermarkets in the spice aisle.

Moros y Cristianos

Makes 8 to 10 servings

3/4 pound dried black beans

2 large tomatoes, puréed in a blender

1 large white onion, finely diced

1 cup finely diced celery

1/4 cup extra-virgin olive oil

2 tablespoons minced garlic

1 teaspoon dried marjoram

2 bay leaves

1 1/2 tablespoons sea salt

2 cups basmati rice (see note)

3 cups vegetable broth

1 cup chopped fresh cilantro

1/2 cup Simple Garlic Oil (page 22)

The name of this dish literally means "Moors and Christians," and refers to the combination of black beans and rice—a bit of fairly benign racist Cuban humor. I would have self-censored this blatant politically incorrect moniker, but I found no trace of racism (or even class discrimination) while I was in Cuba, so I saw no need to whitewash it (no pun intended) with a made-up substitute name. As is the case in Cuban society, where interracial marriage is a nonissue, the beans and rice are happily mixed in one tasty melting pot. *Ehh-bony aaand I-voryyy . . .*

Pick over the beans to remove any small stones or other debris. Wash well, drain, and place in a bowl with enough fresh water to cover by about 3 inches. Let soak for 8 to 12 hours.

Drain the beans and place them in a heavy soup pot along with the puréed tomatoes, onion, celery, olive oil, garlic, marjoram, and bay leaves. Add enough cold water to cover by about 2 inches and bring to a boil over medium-high heat. Adjust the heat to maintain a steady simmer, cover, and cook for about 1 hour, or until the beans are tender but still hold their shape. Add 1 tablespoon of the salt and cook over very low heat for 15 to 20 minutes longer.

While the beans are cooking, prepare the rice. Wash it very gently in several changes of cold water, taking care not to break the delicate grains. Keep rinsing the rice until the water runs clear. Drain, place in a bowl, and add fresh water to cover. Let soak for 15 to 20 minutes. Drain again and place in a saucepan with the broth and the remaining ¹⁄₂ tablespoon salt. Bring to a boil, reduce the heat to the lowest setting, cover, and cook for 15 minutes. Remove from the heat and fluff very gently with a rubber spatula.

Once the beans are done, gently fold in the rice, taking care not to break the grains too much. Reheat the dish over very low heat. Remove from the heat and stir in the cilantro and Simple Garlic Oil. Serve at once.

White vs. Brown Basmati

Normally I would recommend the less popular brown basmati, as it is a whole grain, but in this application it just wouldn't work. On the bright side, true basmati is not a totally "white" rice, because it is hand polished and the bran is not fully removed. If you look closely, you'll see traces of it still intact, forming a thin sheath. A small consolation, perhaps, but the difference is palpable in properly cooked basmati; instead of a sticky mush, the grains stand apart, gorgeously elongated and fluffy. True basmati also has an unparalleled aroma—you can smell it cooking a block away. Brown basmati, alas, though more wholesome, has nowhere near the same appeal; the aroma is muddied by the husk's earthy smell. Live a little. Go to an Indian grocery store and ask for Dehraduni basmati rice. If basmati is the king of rice (which it is), then the basmati grown in Dehradun is the emperor.

Pinto Beans
with Scallions and Cilantro

Makes 6 to 8 servings

1 pound dried pinto beans

1 large onion, finely diced

1 green bell pepper, finely diced

2 tablespoons minced garlic

1 tablespoon sea salt

2 to 3 bunches scallions, thinly sliced

1 to 2 bunches cilantro, coarsely chopped

1 cup Simple Garlic Oil (page 22)

*P*ick over the beans to remove any small stones or other debris. Wash well, drain, and place in a bowl with enough fresh water to cover by about 3 inches. Let soak for 8 to 12 hours.

Drain the beans and place them in a heavy soup pot along with the onion, bell pepper, and garlic. Add enough cold water to cover by about 2 inches and bring to a boil over medium-high heat. Adjust the heat to maintain a steady simmer and cook for about 1 hour, or until the beans are tender but still hold their shape. Add the salt and cook for 5 to 10 minutes longer. The liquid should be fairly thick. Stir in the scallions and cilantro. Remove from the heat and stir in the Simple Garlic Oil. Serve at once, in bowls as a side dish or on a plate with rice and vegetables. If you wish, pass a spicy sauce, such as Chipotle Chili Sauce (page 31), separately to give the beans an extra dimension.

This is pretty simple but it's very good. If you like beans, it'll become an instant favorite, guaranteed.

Alternatively, the beans may be cooked in a slow cooker for 8 to 12 hours. This eliminates the need to be around to check on them, stir occasionally, and all that.

Quinoa Pilaf

Makes 6 to 8 servings

See photo facing page 97

2 tablespoons extra-virgin olive oil

1 large onion, diced

4 stalks celery, strings removed and diced

1 tablespoon minced garlic

1 green bell pepper, diced

1 yellow bell pepper, diced

1 red bell pepper, diced

2 bunches scallions, sliced

2 zucchini, diced

2 carrots, grated

1 cup quinoa (see note, page 79), well washed and drained

2 cups carrot juice or vegetable broth

1 teaspoon sea salt

1/4 teaspoon freshly ground black pepper

1/2 cup Udo's Oil

1/4 cup chopped fresh parsley

*H*eat the olive oil in a large, heavy pot and add the onion, celery, and garlic, stirring constantly. As soon as the mixture is hot, add the bell peppers and continue stirring. When the mixture has heated through (but is not sizzling), add half the scallions and all of the zucchini, carrots, and quinoa and stir well. Add the carrot juice, salt, and pepper, and stir until well combined. Bring to a simmer, adjust the heat to medium, cover, and cook for about 15 minutes, or until the juice has been absorbed and the quinoa is tender. Remove from the heat and stir in the remaining scallions and the Udo's Oil. Garnish with the parsley and serve at once.

This is a delicious dish, providing complete protein, a varied complement of vegetables, and all your essential fatty acids in one shot. The carrot juice adds both color and a delicious sweetness, but if you prefer, feel free to substitute vegetable broth. Either way, this is a crowd-pleaser.

Whole Spelt Baked in Kabocha Squash

Makes 4 to 8 servings

1 cup spelt berries

4 cups water or vegetable broth

1 teaspoon sea salt

2 kabocha squashes (about 2 pounds each)

1½ cups freshly grated Parmesan cheese

1 cup finely diced red onion

1 cup finely diced celery

4 cloves garlic, peeled, crushed, and finely minced

¼ teaspoon freshly ground black pepper

½ cup Udo's Oil

1 tablespoon chopped fresh parsley

*C*over the spelt berries with water and soak overnight. Drain and place in a saucepan with the water and ½ teaspoon of the salt. Bring to a boil, reduce the heat to maintain a gentle, low simmer, cover, and cook until the grains are tender but chewy, about 1 hour and 20 minutes. If any liquid remains, raise the heat to high and cook until the spelt berries are almost dry.

Cut into the tops of the squashes at an inward angle to remove a "lid" section around the stem. Scrape out the seeds and stringy inner walls. Sprinkle the inside of the squashes with salt and pepper.

Preheat the oven to 350 degrees F. Combine the spelt with the Parmesan cheese, onion, celery, garlic, the remaining salt, and the pepper and stir until thoroughly combined. Taste and adjust the seasonings, if needed.

Spelt is a little-known grain used primarily as an alternative to wheat by people with wheat sensitivities. It has an agreeable nutty flavor that goes well with Parmesan cheese (almost anything does) and blends nicely with virtually all vegetables, especially when it is baked in a squash. This is a great finished dish to take camping for your first night out, when it's enough hassle just to pitch the tent, set up camp, and build a fire. Simply wrap the cooked squashes in foil and stick them in the fire for a little while to reheat.

Stuff the squashes with the spelt mixture. Replace the "lids," sealing the mixture inside the squashes. Place them on a baking sheet (lined with foil or parchment paper for the easiest cleanup) and bake for about $1\frac{1}{2}$ hours, or until the squash is tender.

To serve, remove the "lids" and cut the squashes in halves or quarters. Place on plates and drizzle each serving with some of the Udo's Oil. Sprinkle with the parsley and serve at once.

VEGETABLES

There is simply no limit to the wealth of diverse colors, shapes, textures, and sheer explosion of flavors provided by the world of vegetables. It is plant life that gives food real depth and character and brings us hot, sour, pungent, and bitter tastes. No dish of any sophistication exists without the presence of vegetables, and any number of complex vegetable dishes can be made with no animal-based ingredients whatsoever. Furthermore, the nutrients provided by animal products are all available from plant sources. Add this up and you have an excellent argument for a vegetarian diet, even before throwing into the equation such issues as food cost, the negative impact of animal farming on the environment, health problems arising from the consumption of animal products, or any of the ethical and religious arguments against the exploitation, mistreatment, and killing of sentient beings.

Of course, none of these abstract reasons need to be considered in order to appreciate the bounty of the vegetable kingdom. All you really need is a nose and a mouth. Vegetables are to food what color and sound are to the movies.

Artichoke Purée

Makes 4 servings

6 large globe artichokes

1 large lemon

2 tablespoons freshly squeezed lemon juice

4 cloves garlic, peeled and crushed

1 bay leaf

1 tablespoon whole fennel seeds

1 teaspoon whole black peppercorns

1 tablespoon sea salt, plus more as needed

1 tablespoon butter

¼ cup Udo's Oil

1 tablespoon snipped chives (optional)

*P*ut the artichokes in a large pot and fill it with water to within 2 inches of the top. Take out the artichokes and bring the water to a boil. While the water is heating, remove and discard the outer leaves from the artichokes. Cut the lemon in half and use the halves to rub lemon juice onto the exposed flesh of the artichokes as you work, to keep them from discoloring. Pare away the tough outer portion of the artichoke bottoms, leaving only the white flesh— again, rub with the lemon as you go to keep the flesh from discoloring.

Add the artichokes, the used lemon halves, 1 tablespoon of the lemon juice, and the garlic, bay leaf, fennel seeds, peppercorns, and salt to the boiling water. When the water returns to a boil, turn down the heat to maintain a steady simmer and cook until the artichokes are very tender, at least 30 minutes. Test with a fork; they should pierce easily.

Remove the artichokes with a slotted spoon and drain well. Gently push off the remaining leaves and the hairy choke, leaving only the meaty hearts. Place the hearts in a food processor with the butter and the remaining 1 tablespoon lemon juice and process until smooth. Taste and add more salt, if needed. Keep warm in a bowl set over hot (not boiling) water until ready to serve.

To serve, whisk the artichoke purée and add the oil, whisking to blend it in well. Serve in a bowl, as part of a buffet, or on individual plates, garnished with the chives, if using.

This was my son's first solid food. I served it at my wedding, too, alongside porcini mushrooms. It's a smooth-as-silk comfort food, rich tasting yet light and airy. And it's a lot easier to make than anyone might think from looking at the prickly things.

Asparagus with Spicy Vinaigrette

Makes 4 servings

1 pound asparagus, washed and trimmed

3 tablespoons Udo's Oil

2 small shallots, finely diced

1 tablespoon balsamic vinegar

1 tablespoon brown rice vinegar

2 teaspoons Sriracha Sauce (page 38)

½ teaspoon ground cumin, lightly toasted

¼ teaspoon sea salt

¼ teaspoon freshly ground black pepper

1 tablespoon finely slivered scallion

Steam the asparagus until tender-crisp. While the asparagus is steaming, combine the oil, shallots, balsamic vinegar, brown rice vinegar, Sriracha Sauce, cumin, salt, and pepper to compose the vinaigrette. Divide the asparagus spears among 4 plates, facing them all in the same direction, forming attractive piles. Whisk the vinaigrette lightly and pour artfully over the asparagus. Garnish with the scallion. Serve warm or at room temperature.

Asparagus is a kingly vegetable. With this fiery sauce, it becomes a *warrior* king, asserting its presence fiercely on the palate. This is an excellent appetizer, due as much to its restrained quantity as to the way one literally reaches for the next dish to mollify the sting of the vinaigrette.

Baby Bok Choy with Curry Oil

Makes 4 servings

8 baby bok choy
¼ cup Curry Oil (page 24)
¼ teaspoon sea salt
¼ teaspoon freshly ground black pepper

*T*rim the root ends of the bok choy and cut a deep X in the bottom with the point of a paring knife. Wash well. Bring a large pot of salted water to a boil. Drop in the bok choy, pushing it under the water with a spoon. Wait about 1 minute, then lift the bok choy out with a slotted spoon and lay them on a towel. Be careful keep them in their original shape as much as possible. Working quickly, arrange the bok choy on heated plates, drizzle with the Curry Oil, and sprinkle with the salt and pepper. Serve at once.

> You can also add a light drizzle of Chili Oil (page 23) for added spice and color contrast. If the bok choy seems a little too chewy for your taste, just cook it a bit longer. However, be aware that the green part will soften much sooner than the root end, and it will most likely be preferable to have a chewier stem over mushy leaves. Be careful how you manage the trade-off.

This recipe is both easy and elegant. When shopping, look for baby bok choy with very bright, healthy green leaves.

Beets and Broccoli Stems

Makes 4 to 6 servings

    3 medium to large beets
    6 to 8 large broccoli stems
    1/4 cup Simple Garlic Oil (page 22)
    1/2 teaspoon sea salt
    1/4 teaspoon freshly ground black pepper

Peel the beets and broccoli stems and cut them into medium dice. Toss them together and place them in a steamer. Steam for 10 to 15 minutes, or until the beets are tender (the broccoli stems will be a bit softer). Toss the vegetables in a bowl with the Simple Garlic Oil, salt, and pepper. Serve at once.

Stop throwing away those thick broccoli stems. They're actually quite good in other dishes, including vegetable soup, and they have all the same good stuff in them as the tops. Here's a marvelous dish that brings out the best in both broccoli stems and beets—and as you'll see, it's very quick and easy to make. If you're one of those health freak purists, you can scrub the skins and leave them on instead of peeling them.

Bitter Melon with Ginger

Makes 4 servings

4 medium bitter melons
1 piece (2 inches) fresh ginger
1 red onion, diced
4 large ripe tomatoes, grated
1 cup vegetable broth
1 tablespoon ground coriander
1 tablespoon garam masala (see note, page 145)
1 teaspoon turmeric
1 teaspoon cayenne
1/4 cup Udo's Oil

Split the bitter melons in half lengthwise and scrape out the seeds with the tip of a spoon. Slice them on the diagonal, about 1/2 inch thick. Peel the ginger and slice it crosswise about 1/4 inch thick. With the back of a wooden spoon, mash the ginger slices slightly. Combine all the ingredients except the Udo's Oil in a heavy saucepan and bring to a simmer. Adjust the heat to maintain a steady simmer, cover, and cook until the bitter melon is tender, about 30 minutes or longer. The tomatoes and broth should be reduced to a thick, creamy sauce. Remove from the heat, stir in the oil, and serve at once.

This is a good way for the fainthearted to try bitter melon for the first time. The tomato tames the bitterness, and the spices make it taste more like a familiar curry than some freaky exotic thing. Serve this with aromatic basmati rice and a simple steamed green.

Brazilian-Style Blanched Collard Greens

Makes 4 servings

You'll need a sharp knife for this. Once you get the collards washed and cut, the rest is easy. And it's really good—and good for you, too.

¼ cup Simple Garlic Oil (page 22)
½ teaspoon crushed red chiles
½ teaspoon sea salt
¼ teaspoon freshly ground black pepper
1 to 2 bunches (depending on their size) very fresh collard greens

Combine the Simple Garlic Oil, crushed red chiles, salt, and pepper in a small bowl and mix with a wooden spoon, bruising the chile pieces as much as possible to release their flavor and aroma. Set aside to allow the flavors to develop.

Wash the collard leaves thoroughly and pat dry. Cut out the center ribs. Stack several leaves in a pile and slice them crosswise to make very thin shreds. Repeat with the remaining leaves.

Bring a large pot of salted water to a boil. Drop in the collard greens, pushing them under the water with a spoon. Wait about 1 minute, then drain the leaves in a colander. Press down with the back of the spoon to squeeze as much of the water out as possible. Transfer to a bowl and toss with the oil mixture. Serve at once.

If the greens are a bit too chewy for your taste, just cook them a little while longer.

Carrots, Burdock, and Hijiki

Makes 4 to 6 servings

1/2 pound carrots, well scrubbed and julienned diagonally

1/2 pound burdock root (see note, page 139), well scrubbed and julienned diagonally

2 ounces hijiki, rinsed and soaked in fresh water to cover until reconstituted (about 20 minutes)

1/2 cup vegetable broth

1/4 cup soy sauce

2 tablespoons sake

2 tablespoons mirin (see note, page 139)

1/4 teaspoon sea salt

1/4 cup Udo's Oil

*P*reheat the oven to 375 degrees F. Combine the carrots, burdock root, hijiki, broth, soy sauce, sake, mirin, and salt in a heavy, ovenproof saucepan. Bring to a simmer over high heat. Cover tightly and place in the oven. Roast for about 1 hour, or until the vegetables are tender (the burdock will remain a little fibrous). Check every 20 minutes to make sure enough liquid remains to prevent the vegetables from browning. If necessary, add water, a little at a time, checking more often near the end.

Remove from the oven and return to the stove (be very careful not to burn yourself, as the handle of the pan will be hot!). Cook a few minutes to reduce the juices to a few tablespoons, stirring constantly. Remove from the heat, stir in the oil, and serve at once.

For anyone who missed the hippie period, this was one of the popular comfort foods of the time. Eat it with brown rice for the full effect. Hijiki (also called hiziki), if you don't already know, is a variety of dried seaweed, available from Japanese and natural food markets. If the hijiki tastes too briny to you, try soaking it in apple or pineapple juice. Try to pick carrots that are about the same thickness as the burdock root, which will ensure uniform cooking and a more eye-appealing result.

Photo: Chocolate-Mint Mousse (page 184)

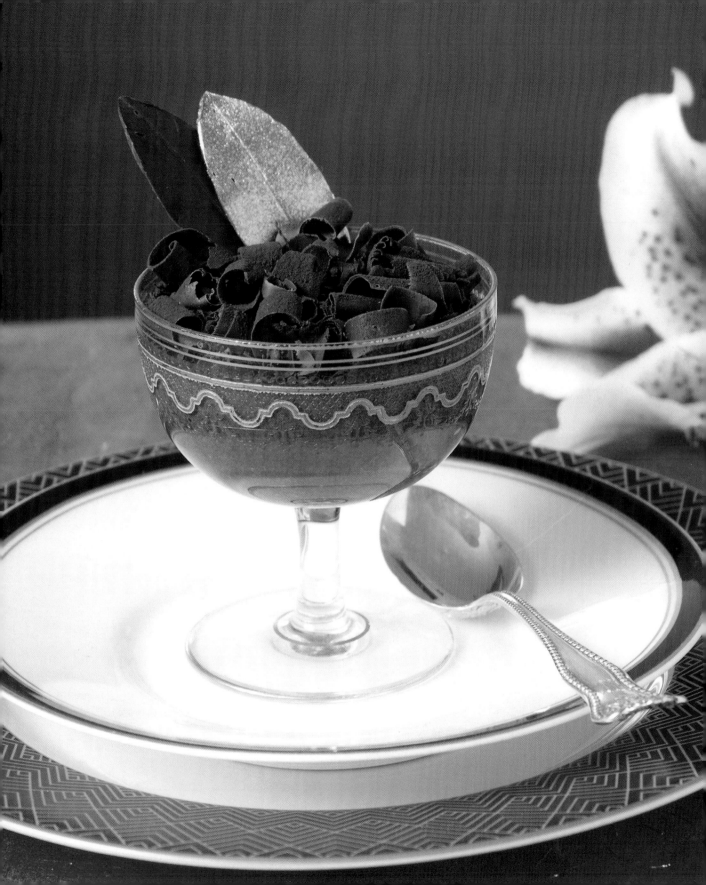

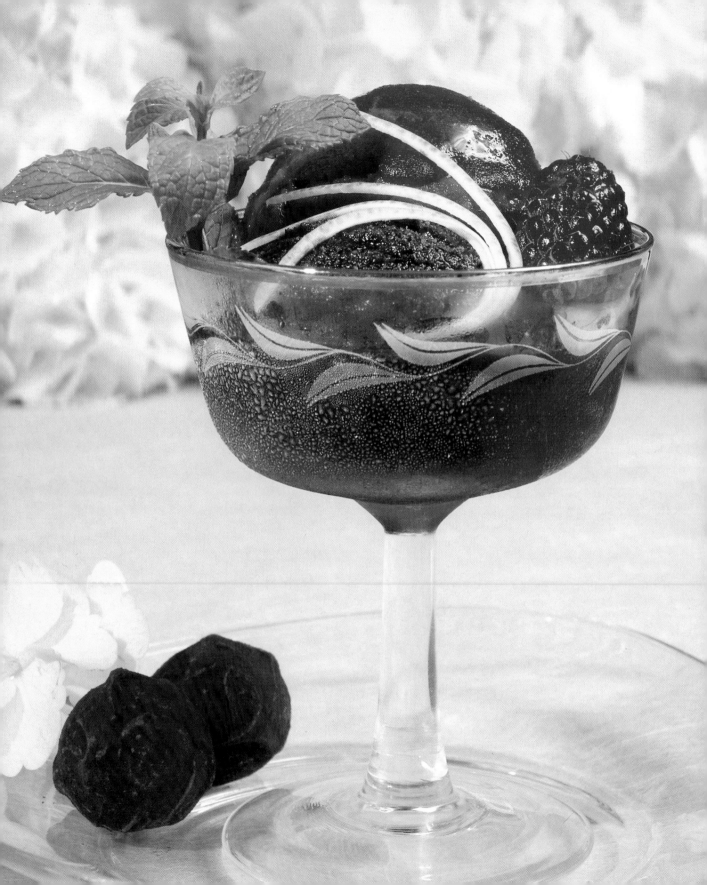

Cauliflower with Olives, Peppers, and Parsley

Makes 4 to 6 servings

1 large head cauliflower, separated into florets

1 red bell pepper, roasted (see note, page 26) and finely diced

1/2 cup pitted kalamata olives, finely diced

1/3 cup Simple Garlic Oil (page 22)

2 tablespoons coarsely chopped fresh parsley

1 tablespoon freshly squeezed lemon juice (optional)

1/2 teaspoon sea salt

1/2 teaspoon freshly ground black pepper

Steam the cauliflower until tender. Remove the steamer insert and shake gently, allowing any excess water to drain well. Pile up the florets on a plate or platter to reconstruct the original head shape. Combine the roasted pepper, olives, Simple Garlic Oil, 1 tablespoon of the parsley, the optional lemon juice, and the salt and pepper. Spoon over the "head of cauliflower," covering it well and allowing the mixture to trickle down into the interior. Sprinkle with the remaining 1 tablespoon parsley.

The great thing about this dish, aside from the remarkable taste contrasts, is its appearance. The florets are reassembled into what looks like a whole head of cauliflower, then festooned with olives, roasted pepper, and parsley bits. Imagine it on a silver platter, like a work of modern art.

Photo: Goji-Raspberry Sorbet (page 171)

Chayotes with Nutmeg

Makes 4 servings

- 4 chayotes
- 2 tablespoons agave nectar
- 1 tablespoon butter
- 1 teaspoon finely chopped fresh parsley
- 1/2 teaspoon freshly grated nutmeg
- 1/2 teaspoon sea salt
- 1/4 teaspoon freshly ground black pepper
- 2 tablespoons Udo's Oil

Place the chayotes in a pot with water to cover and bring to a boil. Reduce the heat to maintain a steady simmer, cover, and cook until they are tender, about 20 minutes. Drain and immediately plunge into ice water to stop the cooking completely. When cool enough to handle, peel the chayotes and remove the tough inner core. There is a delicious almondlike seed in the center, which you must eat. Go ahead—I've never seen the seed included in any dish, so clearly the cook always does this. I always do. Must be some kind of unspoken tradition.

Cut the chayotes into attractive cubes or slices and return them to the pot along with the agave nectar, butter, parsley, nutmeg, salt, and pepper. Warm over low heat, stirring gently to combine well. Remove from the heat, add the oil, and shake the pot to mix it in thoroughly. Serve at once.

Chayotes are a pale green variety of squash, shaped like slightly flattened pears. They're reputed to be highly nutritious and are featured prominently in the bland diet served in Mexican hospitals. I should know—I did hard time in one after a car accident. I was fed a ton of chayotes, but unfortunately they weren't anything like these.

Low-Carb Paglia e Fieno

Makes 8 servings

8 young green zucchini
8 young yellow zucchini
2 tablespoons sea salt
3 tablespoons water
1 tablespoon extra-virgin olive oil
3½ cups Raw Tomato Sauce (page 36)
1 tablespoon julienned fresh basil

*C*ut the ends off the green and yellow zucchini. Using a mandoline or a very sharp knife, cut the zucchini lengthwise into long, very thin julienne. Sprinkle the zucchini with the salt and gently toss. Place in a colander and allow to drain for at least 30 minutes. Once the zucchini are limp and pliable, rinse to remove the excess salt, drain thoroughly, and set aside until serving time.

To serve, heat the water and oil in a large saucepan. When barely simmering, add the zucchini and toss until just heated through. Immediately drain and toss with the Raw Tomato Sauce. Garnish with the basil and serve at once.

The classic Italian dish paglia e fieno, which means "hay and straw," is a combination of fresh yellow and green noodles, normally served in a creamy sauce. Here is a dish inspired by that idea, but without the refined white flour, cholesterol, and all the wrong fats.

This dish can also be served as a salad by omitting the reheating procedure. If desired, a squeeze of fresh lemon juice may be added.

Suffering Succotash

Makes 8 servings

1 red onion, diced

7 cloves garlic, peeled, crushed, and minced

1 red bell pepper, roasted (see note, page 26) and diced

1 green bell pepper, roasted (see note, page 26) and diced

1 tablespoon extra-virgin olive oil

1 pound frozen white corn, cooked

1 pound frozen lima beans, cooked

1/2 teaspoon sea salt

1/2 teaspoon freshly ground black pepper

1 cup Chipotle Mayonnaise (page 58)

1 tablespoon chopped fresh parsley

Place the onion, garlic, peppers, and oil in a large, heavy pot and stir well. Add 2 to 3 tablespoons water and place over high heat until bubbling. Turn the heat down to medium-low, cover, and cook gently until the onion is soft, about 15 minutes. Add a little more water, if needed, to keep the vegetables from browning. Add the corn and lima beans and heat thoroughly. Season with the salt and pepper to taste.

Just before serving, remove from the heat, add the Chipotle Mayonnaise and parsley, and stir well. Serve at once.

Named before its time by Sylvester, the lisping "puddy tat" of Tweety fame, this dish came into being just because I always wanted to make something I could call "suffering succotash."

Gingered Brussels Sprouts

Makes 4 to 6 servings

1 pound very fresh Brussels sprouts

1 piece (1 inch) fresh ginger, peeled, sliced, and cut
    into very thin julienne

1 tablespoon freshly squeezed lime juice

1/4 cup Udo's Oil

1/2 teaspoon sea salt

1/4 teaspoon freshly ground black pepper

*Q*uarter the Brussels sprouts lengthwise and trim away any discolored outer leaves. Place the ginger in a small dish, add the lime juice, and toss well. Blanch the Brussels sprouts in boiling salted water until they are just tender-crisp (no longer than that!). Drain them well and shake them in a colander to remove excess water. Immediately return them to the pot and add the ginger, lime juice, oil, salt, and pepper. Shake the pot vigorously in a circular motion, mixing everything well. Serve immediately.

I always hated Brussels sprouts when I was a kid, only to discover later that this was because everyone always overcooked them to the point where they smelled like old socks and had an unnaturally mushy texture. Here's how to do it right—finally!

Vegetable Lasagne

Makes 6 to 8 servings

Recipe featured on the cover

2 small zucchini, thinly sliced lengthwise

2 yellow zucchini or other yellow summer squash,
    thinly sliced lengthwise

1$\frac{1}{2}$ tablespoons sea salt

1 tablespoon butter

1 large butternut squash (at least 3 pounds)

4 large globe artichokes

2 lemons, cut in half

4 cloves garlic, peeled and crushed

1 teaspoon whole fennel seeds

1 bay leaf

$\frac{1}{2}$ teaspoon whole black peppercorns

2 portobello mushrooms

$\frac{1}{4}$ cup dry Marsala wine or sherry

2 tablespoons chopped shallots

1 tablespoon extra-virgin olive oil

$\frac{1}{2}$ teaspoon freshly ground black pepper

2 red bell peppers, roasted (see note, page 26) and
    cut into 1-inch-wide strips

2 yellow bell peppers, roasted (see note, page 26) and
    cut into 1-inch-wide strips

2 green bell peppers, roasted (see note, page 26) and
    cut into 1-inch-wide strips

1 cup freshly grated Parmesan cheese

$\frac{1}{2}$ to 1 cup Roasted Garlic Purée (page 37)

$\frac{1}{4}$ cup Basil Oil (page 22)

Chopped fresh parsley

Thin slices of butternut squash replace the traditional lasagna noodles in this extraordinary presentation. The Parmesan cheese in this dish is not gratuitous—just enough for flavor. Vegans can enjoy the lasagne with their favorite soy version in its place.

*T*oss the green and yelow zucchini slices with 1 tablespoon of the salt, and set in a colander to drain.

Peel the butternut squash, cut off the round part containing the seeds (reserve it for another use), and cut the remaining squash lengthwise into thin sheets (like lasagne noodles), no more than $1/8$ inch thick. A mandoline is perfect for this. Blanch the sheets in boiling salted water for 15 seconds, plunge into ice water to stop the cooking completely, drain, and dry on towels.

Snap off and discard the outer leaves of each artichoke to expose the heart. With a sharp knife, cut off the stem, making it flush with the bottom of the artichoke, and trim away the tough, fibrous outer flesh. Rub it with the cut side of the lemons as you proceed to prevent discoloration.

Bring about 4 cups of water to a boil with 1 teaspoon of the salt and the garlic, fennel seeds, bay leaf, and peppercorns. Squeeze the juice from the lemons into the water, drop in the lemons, and add the artichokes. Return to a boil, adjust the heat to maintain a steady simmer, cover, and cook for about 25 minutes, or until the artichoke bottoms are tender-crisp. Drain, refresh under cold water, and place on a towel to drain fully. As soon as the artichokes are cool enough to handle, pull off the remaining leaves and carefully scoop out the choke. Rinse away any hairy bits that may cling to them, place the artichoke hearts in a steamer, and steam until just tender, about 30 minutes.

Slice the portobello mushrooms about $1/4$ inch thick, and cut the slices into $1/2$-inch lengths. Put in a sauté pan with the wine, shallots, olive oil, the remaining $1/2$ teaspoon salt, and the pepper. Toss gently, cover, and place over high heat. As soon as the liquid in the pan begins to simmer, uncover the pan. Stir constantly until all the liquid has been absorbed and the mushrooms are tender, about 5 minutes. Transfer to a bowl and set aside.

recipe continues on next page

Combine the peppers in a bowl and toss them together. Thinly slice the artichoke hearts. Rinse the zucchini slices thoroughly under running water; drain, and pat dry with a towel.

Preheat the oven to 375 degrees F. Line an 8-inch-square baking dish with parchment paper. Grease the parchment lightly with the butter.

Trim the butternut squash to fit into the bottom of the prepared baking dish and arrange some of the slices in a tight, single layer, slightly overlapping them. Sprinkle one-third of the mushrooms over the squash, place one-third of the pepper strips and zucchini slices over the mushrooms, and top with one-third of the artichoke slices. Season with salt and pepper and sprinkle one-third of the Parmesan cheese over the top. Repeat the layers 2 more times, ending with a layer of the butternut squash.

Cover with a sheet of buttered parchment paper and place a tight-fitting pan or flat lid on top. Place a weight on the lid to compress the layers. In order to prevent the edges of the casserole from burning, make a moat by placing the baking pan in a larger pan and fill the outer pan with boiling water, to within 1 inch of the rim. Place the entire assembly into the preheated oven and bake for 2 hours. Remove from the oven and let the casserole rest for about 10 minutes before cutting.

To serve, remove the cover, peel away the top parchment paper, and cut into 6 to 8 pieces. Using a metal spatula, carefully transfer to plates. Place a dollop of the Roasted Garlic Purée on top of each serving. Drizzle the Basil Oil over and around each piece, garnish with chopped parsley, and serve at once.

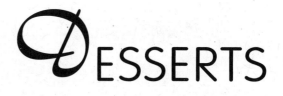ESSERTS

Eating dessert is probably a habit you should avoid, and instead reserve it only for special occasions. (On the other hand, the word "should" has a distinct moralizing tone, which I deplore, so please ignore that last statement if you wish.) I like to think of dessert not as food but as a drug—you don't eat it for your health; you do it for fun. That said, here we go.

I've worked with some of my old favorites to come up with a chapter of desserts that, knowing full well they will be consumed for fun, do the least amount of damage possible and actually offer some health benefits.

As mentioned earlier in this book, chocolate is good for you. If you combine it with healthful ingredients, such as Udo's Oil, there's no reason to suppose that the result will be anything but healthful. So there.

Chocolate and cocoa have finally begun to be recognized as healthful foods (which I've been saying for years, with no scientific evidence to back up my claims). Cacao is very high in antioxidants and other valuable compounds, including flavonoids, which in addition to their antioxidant properties, are also anti-inflammatory and antiviral. This is good news to chocolate lovers, but it's important to note that the healthful properties are associated only with dark chocolate, especially chocolate with a cacao solids content of 70 percent or higher. Milk chocolate has a much lower cacao content and much more sugar; it also contains added dairy solids. Most American chocolate products (no names mentioned) should not be considered healthful, primarily because of the other ingredients in them. Read the labels—it's all junk. Chocolate didn't earn the title "food of the gods" for nothing, so take my advice and don't ever skimp on chocolate quality!

Chocolate-Mint-Banana Sorbet

Makes about 1 quart

6 tablespoons Dutch-process cocoa (preferably Cacao Barry
   Extra Brut or Valrhona)
2 ounces finely chopped bittersweet chocolate
1 cup water
1/2 cup fresh mint leaves, packed and lightly bruised
4 bananas, broken into small pieces
3/4 cup maple syrup
1/4 cup Udo's Oil
1 teaspoon vanilla extract

*P*lace the cocoa and chocolate in a blender. Bring the water
to a boil. Remove from the heat and add the mint. Swirl a
couple of times, and then pour into the blender. Pulse a few
times, and then turn the blender on full speed. Add the
remaining ingredients and continue blending until the mixture is smooth. Strain through a fine mesh sieve into a steel
bowl. Place a sheet of parchment paper directly on the surface of the mixture and allow it to cool. Cover the bowl
tightly and refrigerate until cold.

Remove the mixture from the refrigerator, remove the
parchment paper, and whisk thoroughly. Pour into the work
bowl of an ice cream machine and freeze according to the
manufacturer's instructions. Some ice cream freezers don't
get the sorbet fully firm. If this is the case, scrape the sorbet
into a chilled steel or glass bowl and place it in the freezer for
about 1 hour to finish firming it up. Chill the dishes you plan
to serve the sorbet in. Serve as soon as possible.

Alcohol is unlawful in Morocco, as it is in most Arab countries. So, in Marrakech during the early seventies, young wanderers (like yours truly) would gather in "milk bars," where hashish smoke and rock music filled the air, and the bartenders furiously churned out milkshakes. There were three flavors: chocolate, mint, and banana. You could have them alone or in combination. I tried them all. My favorite (of course) was chocolate-mint-banana.

Goji–Raspberry Sorbet

Makes about 1 quart

See photo facing page 161

6 ounces goji berries
3 cups apple juice
¼ cup agave nectar
¼ cup Udo's Oil
1 pound frozen raspberries, thawed

Soak the goji berries in the apple juice for at least 1 hour, until softened. Purée in a blender until smooth and strain into a bowl. Add the agave nectar and oil. Purée the raspberries lightly, along with any accumulated juice, by short pulses in the blender, taking care not to break up the seeds. Strain through a sieve with mesh just fine enough to catch the seeds, and add the purée to the bowl with the goji berry mixture. Stir well, cover, and refrigerate until cold.

Remove the mixture from the refrigerator and whisk thoroughly. Pour into the work bowl of an ice cream machine and freeze according to the manufacturer's instructions. Some ice cream freezers don't get the sorbet fully firm. If this is the case, scrape the sorbet into a chilled steel or glass bowl and place it in the freezer for about 1 hour to finish firming it up. Chill the dishes you plan to serve the sorbet in. Serve as soon as possible.

Goji berries are well-known in China as a kidney tonic as well as a delicious snack. The best organic berries are sun-dried and packed airtight to preserve both a firm, pliant texture and a sweet, tangy flavor, which is somewhat reminiscent of dried apricots. Since their flavor is a bit foreign to Western palates, they are combined in this recipe with raspberries, which bring the overall taste back to the center.

Goji Sorbet for Purists

If you prefer to make this recipe without the raspberries, just increase the quantity of goji berries to 8 ounces and use 3½ cups apple juice.

Honey-Blueberry Sorbet with Lemon

Makes about 1 quart

4 cups wild blueberries
1⅓ cups honey
½ cup freshly squeezed lemon juice
¼ cup Udo's Oil
2 teaspoons grated lemon zest

Purée the blueberries thoroughly in a blender with the honey, lemon juice, and oil. Pour into a steel or glass bowl and stir in the lemon zest. Cover tightly and refrigerate until cold.

Remove the mixture from the refrigerator and whisk thoroughly. Pour into the work bowl of an ice cream machine and freeze according to the manufacturer's instructions. Some ice cream freezers don't get the sorbet fully firm. If this is the case, scrape the sorbet into a chilled steel or glass bowl and place it in the freezer for about 1 hour to finish firming it up. Chill the dishes you plan to serve the sorbet in. Serve as soon as possible.

This one surprised even me, and I knew what to expect. The blueberry flavor is intense, bespeckled with sudden assertive notes of lemon zest. My twelve-year-old son declared it "the best ever" (a high compliment, believe me).

Mango Sorbet

Makes about 1 quart

3 cups fresh mango chunks (peeled, of course!)
$1/2$ cup water
$1/2$ cup agave nectar
$1/2$ cup freshly squeezed lime juice
$1/4$ cup Udo's Oil
Grated zest of 1 lime

*P*lace all the ingredients in a blender and process until smooth. Strain through a medium-fine mesh sieve to remove any fibrous pulp. Refrigerate until cold.

Remove the mixture from the refrigerator and whisk thoroughly. Pour into the work bowl of an ice cream machine and freeze according to the manufacturer's instructions. Some ice cream freezers don't get the sorbet fully firm. If this is the case, scrape the sorbet into a chilled steel or glass bowl and place it in the freezer for about 1 hour to finish firming it up. Chill the dishes you plan to serve the sorbet in. Serve as soon as possible.

Adding lime juice always brings a fresh spark to mango, awakening its exotic personality. Udo's Oil gives the sorbet a smooth, velvety texture. This is a very rich-tasting dessert, whether served by itself or in a medley of other sorbets.

Tea-Infused Chocolate Sorbet

Makes about 1 quart

2 cups water

4 bags Earl Grey tea

1 cup maple syrup

3/4 cup Dutch-process cocoa (preferably Cacao Barry Extra Brut or Valrhona)

4 ounces finely chopped bittersweet chocolate

1 teaspoon vanilla extract

1/4 cup Udo's Oil

*B*ring the water to a boil. Remove from the heat, add the tea bags, and let steep for about 3 minutes. Remove the tea bags, squeezing gently to extract the last drop of tea. Add the maple syrup and reheat gently (do not boil!). Remove from the heat and add the cocoa, chocolate, and vanilla extract, whisking gently until the cocoa and chocolate have melted completely and the mixture is smooth. Whisk in the oil. Place a sheet of parchment paper directly on the surface of the mixture and let cool. Cover the bowl tightly and refrigerate until cold.

Remove the mixture from the refrigerator, remove the parchment paper, and whisk thoroughly. Pour into the work bowl of an ice cream machine and freeze according to the manufacturer's instructions. Some ice cream freezers don't get the sorbet fully firm. If this is the case, scrape the sorbet into a chilled steel or glass bowl and place it in the freezer for about 1 hour to finish firming it up. Chill the dishes you plan to serve the sorbet in. Serve as soon as possible.

Chocolate sorbet is not an easy thing to make properly. All too often it comes out hard, or grainy, or both. This recipe should work well for you, producing a silky texture because of the oil, which no one else I know of has ever included. Infusing the water with Earl Grey tea gives this sorbet an extra dimension. You can also use any other tea you prefer, or none at all. This recipe will work with or without the tea.

Chocolate sorbet is not as smooth the next day. You'll eat it anyway, of course.

Chocolate Truffles

Truffles, as you probably know, are fungi that grow under the ground near certain trees; they are an epicurean delicacy. In the Périgord, black truffles are hunted out with pigs, which rut and snort around until they locate the secret spot. These chocolate treats got their name because they look vaguely like freshly harvested truffles, round and covered with dirt. Romantic, huh?

Although properly made truffles all look the same on the outside, they may vary widely on the inside. The filling is formed by making a ganache, which is normally a mixture of chocolate and cream to which various flavorings are added. Since we want to use essential fats, we will take a different approach, which, if you have any experience working with chocolate, may shock you. Instead of cream, we'll add water (considered a mortal foe of molten chocolate) and oil (*quelle horreur!*). Believe it or not, it works.

Typically, truffles are served at room temperature, when they're at their creamy best. The wonderful thing about truffles is that it doesn't take many to satisfy that craving for a chocolate treat. Just bite into one and let it slowly melt in your mouth.

Ginger Truffles

Makes about 30 truffles

Ganache
8 ounces dark chocolate, chopped
1 cup water
2 cups peeled and chopped fresh ginger
1/4 cup Udo's Oil
1 tablespoon dark rum (optional)

Chocolate Coating
1/2 cup Dutch-process cocoa (preferably Cacao Barry
Extra Brut or Valrhona)
6 ounces dark chocolate, chopped

To make the ganache, melt the chocolate in a steel bowl set over hot (not boiling) water, stirring occasionally. While the chocolate is melting, place the water and ginger in a small pot and bring to a boil. Lower the heat, cover, and simmer for about 10 minutes. The water should be cloudy with the ginger juice, strongly infused, and reduced by about half. Strain through a fine mesh sieve and measure 1/2 cup. Pour into a clean pot and reheat.

Once the chocolate has melted, whisk in the boiling ginger-infused water, 1 tablespoon at a time. It will seize up at first, but keep whisking and adding the water until it becomes smooth and creamy. Whisk in the oil and optional rum. Cover the bowl and place in the refrigerator for 3 to 4 hours, until firm enough to handle.

Line a tray with parchment or waxed paper. Scoop out 1/2 tablespoon of the chilled ganache for each truffle, form into balls, and place on the tray. Refrigerate until well chilled and firm.

There are many flavors that go well with chocolate. Fresh ginger, like hot chiles, is more than a mere flavor—it's a stimulant, which adds a bright dimension to the chocolate experience as well as an extra flavor layer. Be sure to use a very fine mesh sieve when straining out the chopped ginger so that the ganache will be creamy and smooth, with no distracting fibrous bits.

To make the chocolate coating, line a large tray with parchment or waxed paper. Sift the cocoa evenly over the tray and set aside. Reserve 2 tablespoons of the chocolate and melt the remainder in a steel bowl set over hot (not boiling) water. As soon as the chocolate has melted, remove it from the hot water bath and stir in the 2 tablespoons reserved chocolate. When the chocolate is smooth, remove the ganache balls from the refrigerator.

One by one, dip the ganache balls into the melted chocolate, rolling them between your fingers to coat evenly. Allow the excess to drip back into the bowl and place the coated balls on the tray. Once the chocolate coating has begun to harden, shake the tray gently back and forth to roll the balls in the cocoa, coating them evenly all over. When the coating has fully hardened, lift the truffles off the tray and place them in a container with an airtight lid. Store in the refrigerator until ready to serve. Refrigerated, truffles will keep for about 2 weeks. (Ha! Like that would really happen!) Frozen, they will keep for up to 2 months (only because people won't think to look for them there).

Remove the quantity you want to serve from the refrigerator at least 20 minutes ahead of time to allow the truffles to come to room temperature.

Earl Grey Truffles

Makes about 30 truffles

Ganache
8 ounces dark chocolate, chopped
1/2 cup water
4 bags Earl Grey tea
1 tablespoon honey
1/4 cup Udo's Oil

Chocolate Coating
1/2 cup Dutch-process cocoa (preferably Cacao Barry
    Extra Brut or Valrhona)
6 ounces dark chocolate, chopped

To make the ganache, melt the chocolate in a steel bowl set over hot (not boiling) water, stirring occasionally. While the chocolate is melting, bring the water to a boil in a small saucepan, remove from the heat, and drop in the tea bags and honey. Cover and let steep for 3 to 5 minutes. Remove the tea bags, squeezing gently to extract the liquid.

Once the chocolate has melted, very gently reheat the tea (do not boil!) and whisk it into the chocolate, 1 tablespoon at a time. It will seize up at first, but keep whisking and adding the tea until it becomes smooth and creamy. Whisk in the oil. Cover the bowl and place it in the refrigerator for 3 to 4 hours, until firm enough to handle.

Line a tray with parchment or waxed paper. Scoop out 1/2 tablespoon of the chilled ganache for each truffle, form into balls, and place on the tray. Refrigerate until well chilled and firm.

The French have been using tea in their chocolate recipes for a long time, and for good reason. The subtle floral aroma of tea gives the rich taste of chocolate an elegant background note—in this instance, it is further enhanced by oil of bergamot, the unique flavor in Earl Grey tea.

To make the chocolate coating, line a large tray with parchment or waxed paper. Sift the cocoa evenly over the tray and set aside. Reserve 2 tablespoons of the chocolate and melt the remainder in a steel bowl set over hot (not boiling) water. As soon as the chocolate has melted, remove it from the hot water bath and stir in the 2 tablespoons reserved chocolate. When the chocolate is smooth, remove the ganache balls from the refrigerator.

One by one, dip the ganache balls into the melted chocolate, rolling them between your fingers to coat evenly. Allow the excess to drip back into the bowl and place the coated balls on the tray. Once the chocolate coating has begun to harden, shake the tray gently back and forth to roll the balls in the cocoa, coating them evenly all over. When the coating has fully hardened, lift the truffles off the tray and place them in a container with an airtight lid. Store in the refrigerator until ready to serve. Refrigerated, the truffles will keep for about 2 weeks. (Yeah, right.) Frozen, they will keep for up to 2 months (if you hide them well enough).

Remove the quantity you want to serve from the refrigerator at least 20 minutes ahead of time to allow the truffles to come to room temperature.

Spicy Chocolate-Orange Truffles

Makes about 30 truffles

Ganache
8 ounces dark chocolate, chopped

3/4 cup water

1 teaspoon crushed cardamom seeds (see note, page 74)

1 teaspoon cayenne

2 bay leaves

12 whole black peppercorns

1/4 cup Udo's Oil

1 teaspoon very finely grated orange zest

Chocolate Coating
1/2 cup Dutch-process cocoa (preferably Cacao Barry
     Extra Brut or Valrhona)

6 ounces dark chocolate, chopped

*T*o make the ganache, melt the chocolate in a steel bowl set over hot (not boiling) water, stirring occasionally. While the chocolate is melting, bring the water, cardamom, cayenne, bay leaves, and peppercorns to a boil in a small saucepan. Lower the heat slightly and cook for about 5 minutes, or until reduced to about 3/4 cup. Strain through a very fine mesh sieve to remove all the tiny bits.

Once the chocolate has melted, reheat the water and whisk it into the chocolate, 1 tablespoon at a time. It will seize up at first, but keep whisking and adding the water until it becomes smooth and creamy. Whisk in the oil and orange zest. Cover the bowl and place it in the refrigerator for 3 to 4 hours, until firm enough to handle.

I got the idea of combining chiles with chocolate from the film *Chocolat*. Having grown up in Mexico, this should have happened sooner—I had used them together in savory dishes, but for some reason it didn't occur to me to do this in sweets. Well, that's over—now I use this combination as often as possible, in as many ways as possible. Once you try it, it won't even seem odd to you. The other spices give the truffles a decidedly exotic background; the orange rounds it all out and brings everything together.

Line a tray with parchment or waxed paper. Scoop out $\frac{1}{2}$ tablespoon of the chilled ganache for each truffle, form into balls, and place on the tray. Refrigerate until well chilled and firm.

To make the chocolate coating, line a large tray with parchment or waxed paper. Sift the cocoa evenly over the tray and set aside. Reserve 2 tablespoons of the chocolate and melt the remainder in a steel bowl set over hot (not boiling) water. As soon as the chocolate has melted, remove it from the hot water bath and stir in the 2 tablespoons reserved chocolate. When the chocolate is smooth, remove the ganache balls from the refrigerator.

One by one, dip the ganache balls into the melted chocolate, rolling them between your fingers to coat evenly. Allow the excess to drip back into the bowl and place the coated balls on the tray. Once the chocolate coating has begun to harden, shake the tray gently back and forth to roll the balls in the cocoa, coating them evenly all over. When the coating has fully hardened, lift the truffles off the tray and place them in a container with an airtight lid. Store in the refrigerator until ready to serve. Refrigerated, truffles will keep for about 2 weeks. (Uh-huh.) Frozen, they will keep for up to 2 months (if you live alone, maybe).

Remove the quantity you want to serve from the refrigerator at least 20 minutes ahead of time to allow the truffles to come to room temperature.

Danny's Chocolate Pie

Makes 8 servings

1/4 cup Udo's Oil

19 ounces semisweet chocolate, finely chopped

6 ounces sliced almonds

28 ounces soft silken tofu

3 tablespoons Amaretto liqueur (optional)

2 tablespoons vanilla extract

2 bananas, sliced

1 to 2 tablespoons Dutch-process cocoa

*V*ery lightly oil a 9-inch pie pan with just a few drops of the oil and place it in the refrigerator. Melt 5 ounces of the chocolate in a steel bowl set over hot (not boiling) water. Remove the prepared pie pan from the refrigerator and scatter a few of the almonds over the bottom. Drizzle one-third of the melted chocolate over the almonds and onto the sides of the pie pan, in a random, latticelike pattern, using a small spoon. (If you feel comfortable using a paper cornet, this would be much easier. See note, page 96 for instructions.) Immediately sprinkle one-third of the sliced almonds over the melted chocolate. Press on the almonds lightly to help them adhere. Return the pie pan to the refrigerator for a few minutes. Repeat this process 2 more times, to produce a thin chocolate-almond crust.

I just love it when someone else cooks. One such evening, after dinner, I was presented with this chocolate pie, with no explanation or disclaimer. After I declared it the best part of the meal, I was informed that the main ingredient was in fact tofu. Two words: shock and awe. My version of this pie has few alterations, so I've named it after my good friend, in fond remembrance of an occasion on which I ate well but didn't have to cook.

Melt the remaining 14 ounces chocolate in a stainless steel bowl set over hot (not boiling) water. Place the tofu in a blender with the remaining oil, the optional Amaretto, and the vanilla extract and process until smooth and creamy. With the motor running, add the melted chocolate. Blend until the color is uniform.

Pour a small amount of the tofu mixture over the prepared crust and spread it evenly over the bottom. Arrange half of the banana slices over the mixture. Pour half of the remaining tofu mixture over the banana slices and arrange the remaining banana slices on the surface. Pour on the remainder of the tofu mixture, carefully spreading it to the edge of the pie. Refrigerate for 2 hours. Remove from the refrigerator and dust with the cocoa. Cut with a hot, dry knife.

Chocolate-Mint Mousse

Makes 8 to 12 servings

See photo facing page 160

12 ounces dark chocolate, chopped

10 tablespoons boiling water

$1/2$ cup Udo's Oil

1 teaspoon mint extract

$1/4$ teaspoon peppermint oil

8 egg whites

Pinch of cream of tartar

Chocolate shavings (optional)

*M*elt the chopped chocolate in a stainless steel bowl set over hot (not boiling) water, stirring occasionally. Once it has melted, remove it from the hot water bath and whisk in the boiling water, 1 tablespoon at a time. It will seize up at first, but keep whisking and adding the water until it becomes smooth and creamy. Whisk in the Udo's Oil, mint extract, and peppermint oil.

Whisk the egg whites until foamy, add the cream of tartar, and beat until stiff but not dry. If you prefer, you may use an electric mixer, but be careful not to overbeat. Fold one-quarter of the egg whites into the chocolate mixture to lighten it, and then fold in the rest. This must be done gently but quickly to prevent the mixture from becoming grainy. Pour into 8 to 12 dessert goblets (depending on the size of the goblet) and refrigerate until set, about 4 hours. Garnish with the optional chocolate shavings and serve.

Mint goes well with chocolate, especially when it's served cold. This mousse is utterly simple yet profoundly gratifying. Resist the urge to add whipped cream—it doesn't need any. Use a chocolate composed of at least 65 percent cacao content for the best results. After your guests have begun their spasmodic utterances of blissful approval, you can go ahead and tell them what's in it. Show them the recipe if they don't believe you.

Raw Eggs and Salmonella

If you have any concerns about salmonella in raw eggs, let me assure you first of all that the risk is extremely low. I have been using raw eggs in recipes for over twenty-five years without a single incident. However, your concern is valid, and there are a few things you can do to bring the risk to near zero.

1. Buy refrigerated eggs and keep them refrigerated; salmonella proliferates dangerously at room temperature.

2. Inspect the shells for cracks; salmonella comes from outside the egg, and it can only infect the egg if the integrity of the shell is compromised. Typically, healthy eggs have thick, virtually impenetrable shells, while those sweatshop, hormone-driven, factory-laid eggs have thin, fragile shells.

3. Wash the eggs with warm soapy water and rinse them thoroughly. While you're at it, wash your hands, too.

4. Be scrupulous in using very clean utensils and work surfaces.

5. As soon as you've completed the step in a recipe involving raw eggs, refrigerate the dish and keep it cold until serving time.

6. Relax. A little bacteria is good for your immune system. Ever see babies pick stuff up off the floor and stuff it in their innocent, vulnerable little mouths? We all did it, and we're all still here.

7. If you have a pre-existing immune deficiency, such as HIV, ignore #6. There are some things that aren't worth the risk, even Chocolate-Mint Mousse (page 184).

INDEX

Recipe titles appear in italic typeface.
Page numbers in italics refer to sidebars.

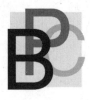

BOOK PUBLISHING COMPANY

since 1974—books that educate, inspire, and empower

To find your favorite vegetarian and soyfood products online, visit:
www.healthy-eating.com

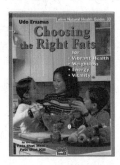

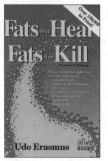

Books by Udo Erasmus

Choosing the Right Fats
978-1-555312-035-3 $11.95

Fats That Heal Fats That Kill
978-0-920470-38-1 $22.95

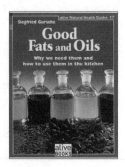

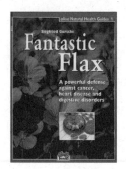

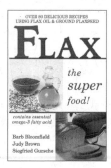

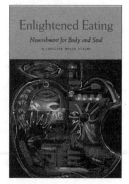

Good Fats and Oils
Siegfried Gursche
978-1-551312-018-6
$11.95

Fantastic Flax
Siegfried Gursche
978-1-55312-000-1
$11.95

Flax the super food
Siegfried Gursche
Barb Bloomfield
Judy Brown
978-1-57067-099-2
$9.95

Enlightened Eating
Caroline Marie Dupont
978-1-55312-041-4 $19.95

Purchase these health titles and cookbooks from your local bookstore
or natural food store, or you can buy them directly from:

Book Publishing Company • P.O. Box 99 • Summertown, TN 38483
1-800-695-2241

Please include $3.95 per book for shipping and handling.